The Vib[illegible]

Desse[illegible] Book

A Complete Collection of Desserts to Start Your Plant-Based Diet and Boost Your Day

Sheryl Ward

Table of Contents

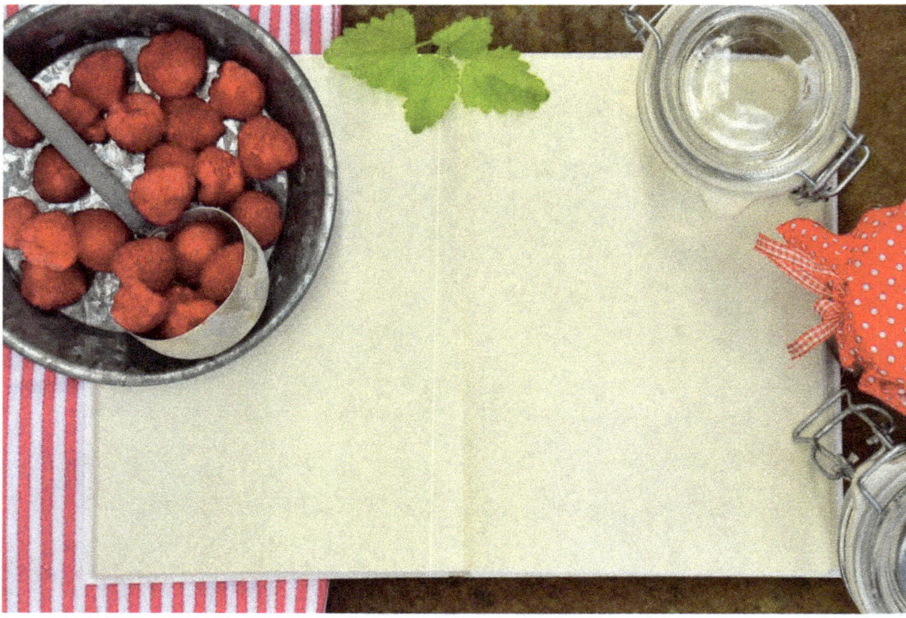

Dark Chocolate Raspberry Ice Cream

Preparation time: 5 minutes Cooking time: 0 minute Servings: 2

Ingredients:

2 frouncesen bananas, sliced ¼ cup fresh raspberries 2 tablespoons cocoa powder, unsweetened 2 tablespoons raspberry jelly

Directions:

Place all the ingredients in a food processor, except for berries and pulse for 2 minutes until smooth. Distribute the ice cream mixture between two bowls, stir in berries until combined, and then serve immediately

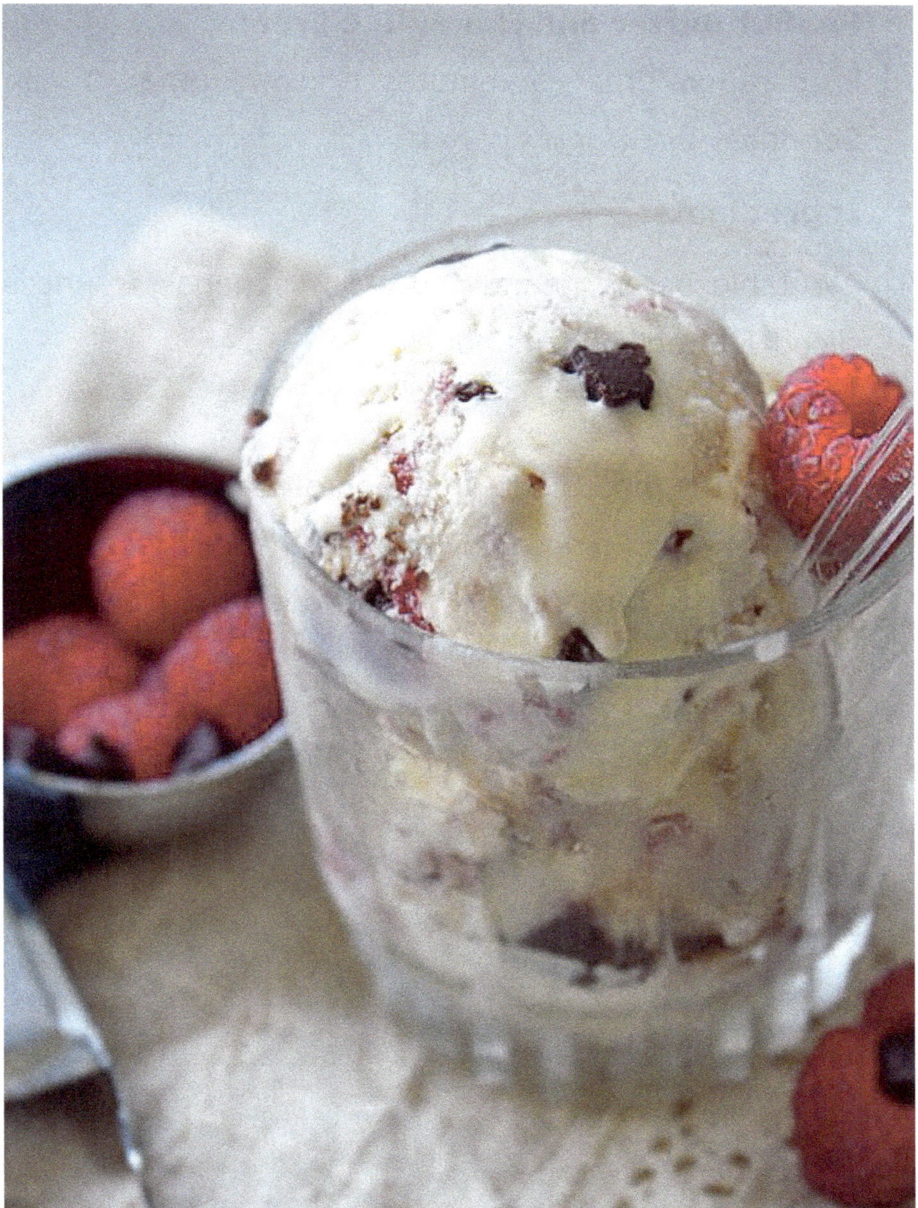

Peanut Butter and Honey Ice Cream

Preparation time: 5 minutes Cooking time: 0 minute Servings: 2

Ingredients:

2½ tablespoons peanut butter 2 bananas frouncesen, sliced 1½ tablespoons honey

Directions:

Place all the ingredients in a food processor and pulse for 2 minutes until smooth. Distribute the ice cream mixture between two bowls and then serve immediately.

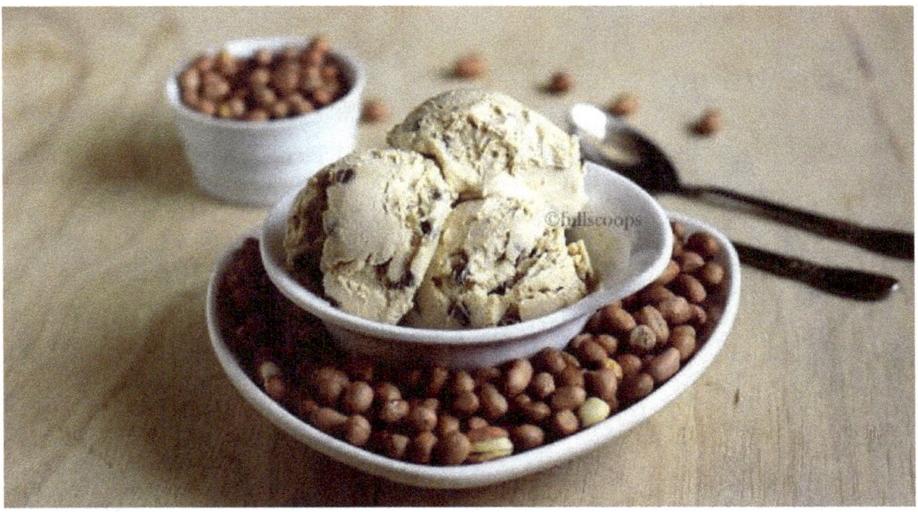

Chocolate Pudding

Preparation time: 5 minutes Cooking time: 0 minute Servings: 4

Ingredients:

3/4 cup cocoa powder 12 ounces tofu, silken 1/3 cup almond milk, unsweetened 1/2 cup sugar Whipped cream for topping

Directions:

Place all the ingredients in a food processor and pulse for 2 minutes until smooth. Distribute the pudding between four bowls, refrigerate for 15 minutes, then top with whipped topping and serve immediately.

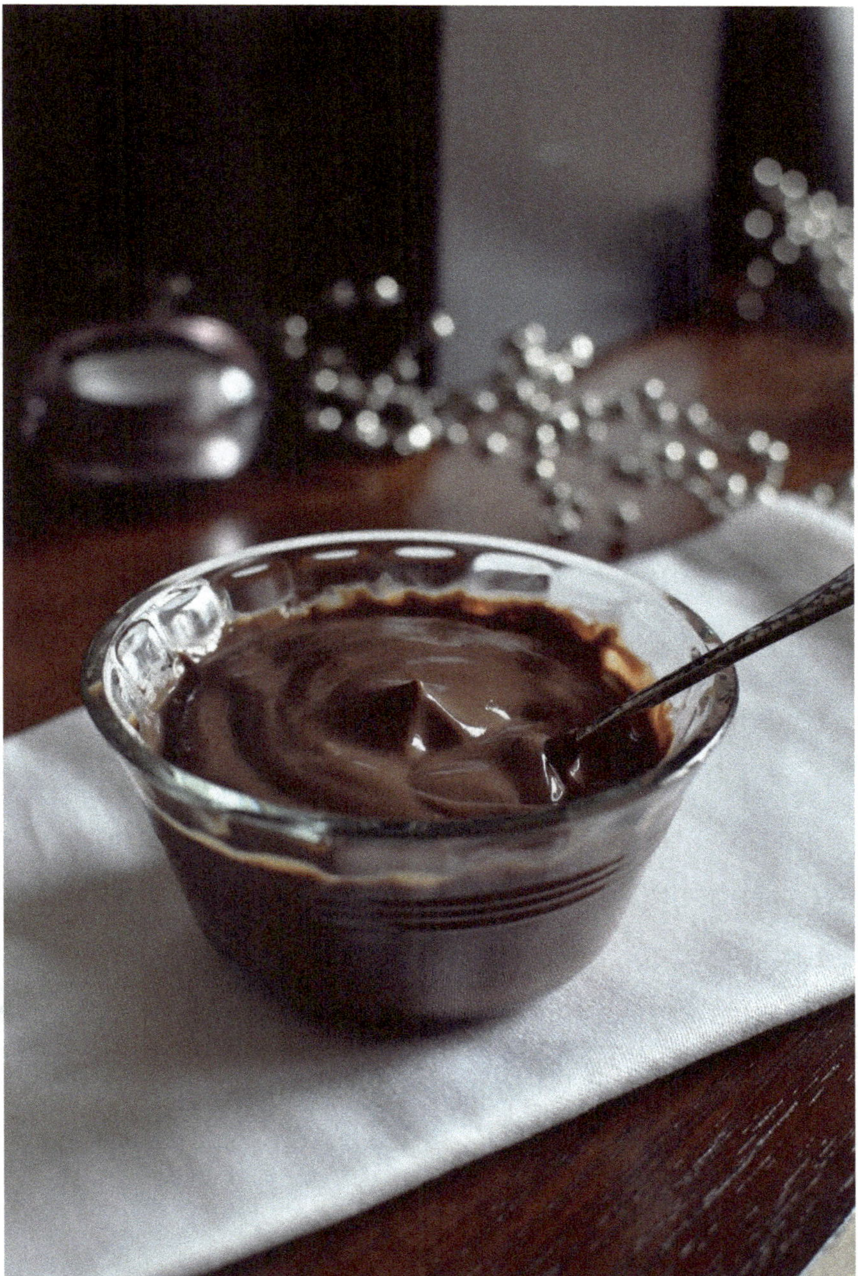

Almond Butter Cookies

Preparation time: 35 minutes Cooking time: 5 minutes Servings: 13

Ingredients:

1/4 cup sesame seeds 1 cup rolled oats 3 Tablespoons sunflower seeds, roasted, unsalted 1/8 teaspoon sea salt 1 1/2 Tablespoons coconut flour 1/2 cup coconut sugar 1/2 teaspoons vanilla extract, unsweetened 3 Tablespoons coconut oil 2 Tablespoons almond milk, unsweetened 1/3 cup almond butter, salted

Directions:

Take a saucepan, place it over medium heat, pour in milk, stir in sugar and oil and bring the mixture to a low boil. Boil the mixture for 1 minute, then remove the pan from heat, and stir in remaining ingredients until incorporated and well combined. Drop the prepared mixture onto a baking sheet lined with wax paper, about 13 cookies, and let the cookies stand for 25 minutes until firm and set. Serve straight away.

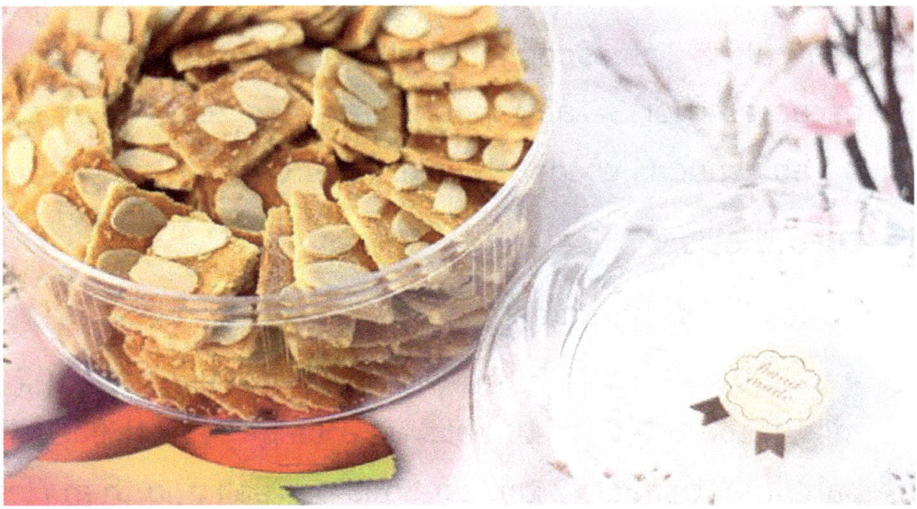

Coconut Cacao Bites

Preparation time:1 hour and 10 minutesCooking time:0 minute Servings: 20

Ingredients:

1 1/2 cups almond flour 3 dates, pitted 1 1/2 cups shredded coconut, unsweetened 1/4 teaspoons ground cinnamon 2 Tablespoons flaxseed meal 1/16 teaspoon sea salt 2 Tablespoons vanilla protein powder 1/4 cup cacao powder 3 Tablespoons hemp seeds 1/3 cup tahini 4 Tablespoons coconut butter, melted

Directions:

Place all the ingredients in a food processor and pulse for 5 minutes until the thick paste comes together. Drop the mixture in the form of balls on a baking sheet lined with parchment sheet, 2 tablespoons per ball and then freeze for 1 hour until firm to touch. Serve straight away

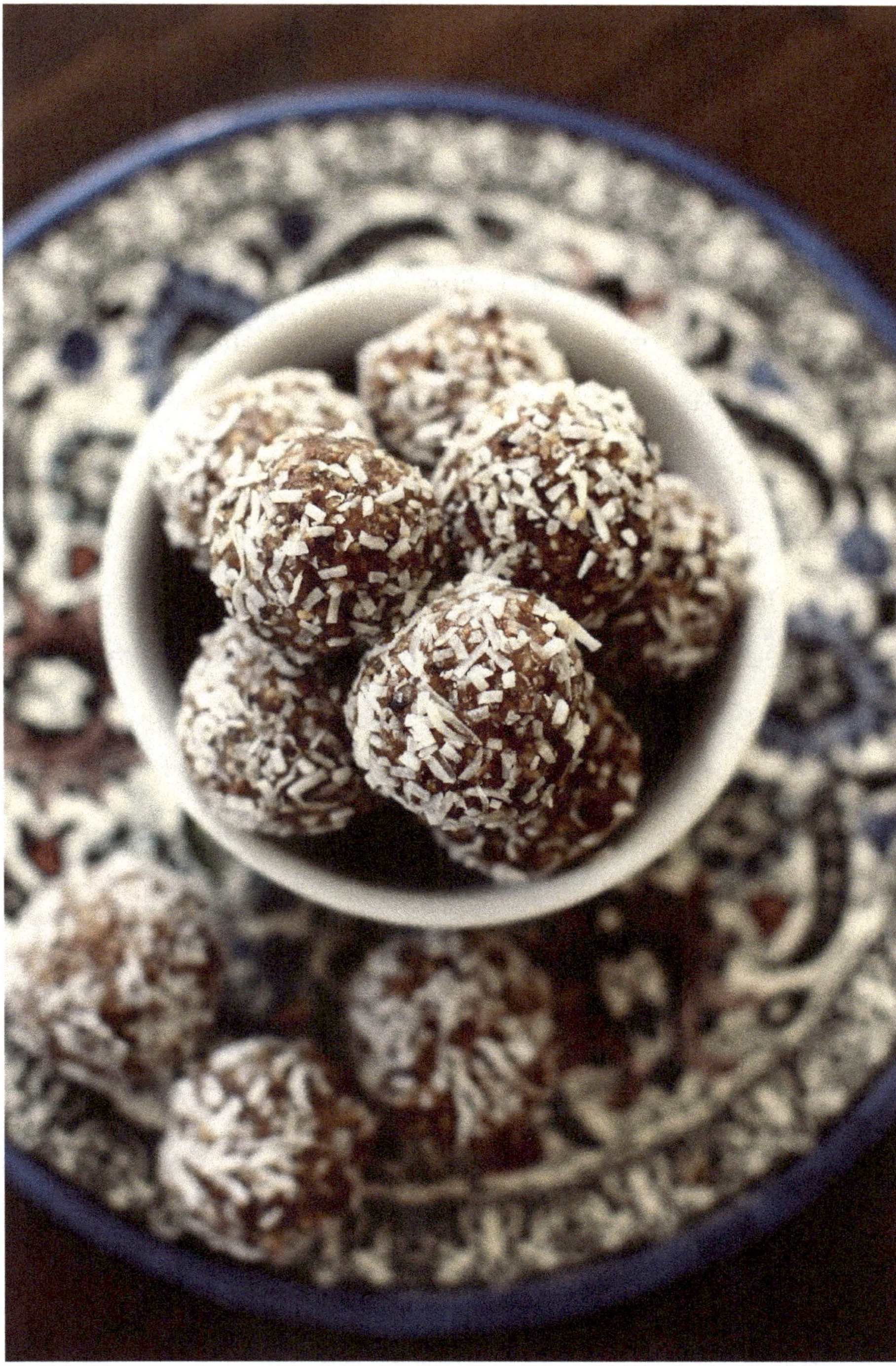

Chocolate Cookies

Preparation time: 40 minutes Cooking time: 5 minutes Servings: 4

Ingredients:

1/2 cup coconut oil 1 cup agave syrup 1/2 cup cocoa powder 1/2 teaspoon salt 2 cups peanuts, chopped 1 cup peanut butter 2 cups sunflower seeds

Directions:

Take a small saucepan, place it over medium heat, add the first three ingredients, and cook for 3 minutes until melted. Boil the mixture for 1 minute, then remove the pan from heat and stir in salt and butter until smooth. Fold in nuts and seeds until combined, then drop the mixture in the form of molds onto the baking sheet lined with wax paper and refrigerate for 30 minutes. Serve straight away.

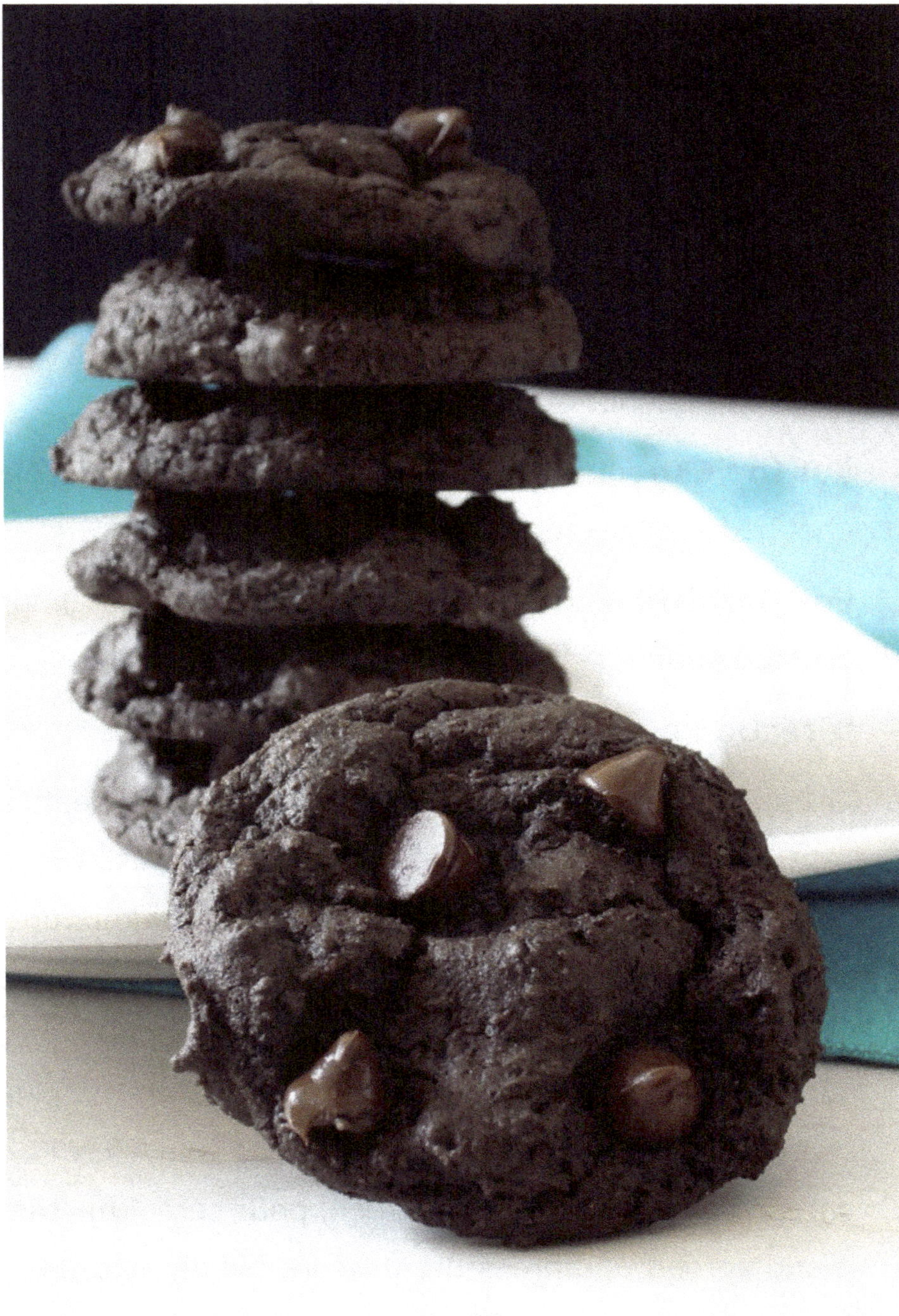

Chocolate Peanut Butter Bars

Preparation time:1 hour and 15 minutes Cooking time:5 minutes Servings: 4

Ingredients:

For the Bars: 2½ cups puffed brown rice cereal ¼ teaspoon salt 1/3 cup maple syrup 2 tablespoons coconut oil ½ cup peanut butter

For the Chocolate Topping: 6 ounces dark chocolate, chopped 2 tablespoons peanut butter

For Garnish: 1 teaspoon flaky sea salt ¼ cup chopped roasted peanuts

Directions:

Take a saucepan, place it over medium-low heat, add salt, butter, coconut oil, and maple syrup, whisk well and bring the mixture to a boil. Then simmer the mixture for 3 minutes, whisking continuously, and remove the pan from heat. Place cereal in a bowl, pour prepared butter syrup over it, and stir until combined and completely coated. Take an 8 by 8 inched baking pan, line it with parchment paper, grease with oil, pour cereal mixture in it and spread and press the mixture evenly and then let the mixture stand for 30 minutes. Prepare the chocolate topping, and for this, place its ingredients in a heatproof bowl and microwave for 2 minutes until chocolate has melted, stirring every 30 seconds. Drizzle chocolate over firmed bars, sprinkle with salt, garnish with peanuts, refrigerate for 30 minutes, then cut it into sixteen bars and serve.

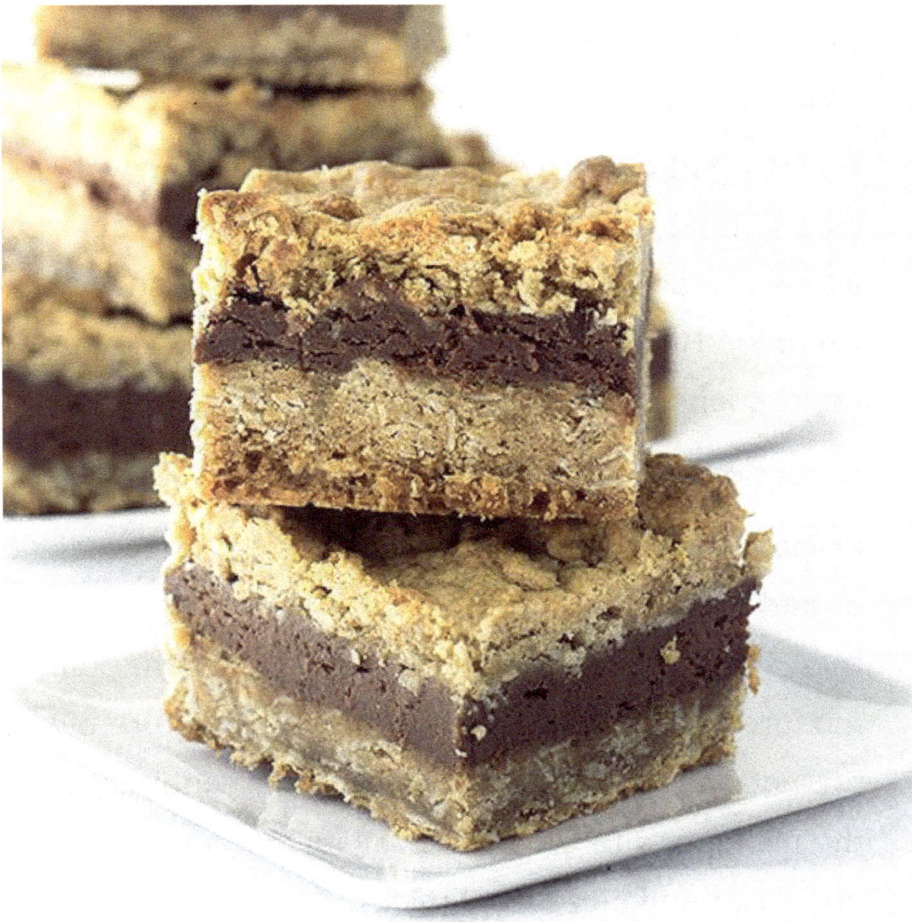

Chocolate Tart

Preparation time:3 hours and 15 minutes Cooking time 0 minute Servings: 8

Ingredients:

For the Crust: 1 cup almonds 2 tablespoons coconut oil ¼ teaspoon agave nectar 3 dates, pitted, soaked in warm water, drained 1 tablespoon cacao powder

For the Filling: 1 1/2 cups of soaked cashews 1/2 cup, plus 2 tablespoons water 1/2 cup, plus 2 tablespoons agave nectar 1/2 cup coconut oil 1/2 teaspoon vanilla 1/4 teaspoon Himalayan pink salt 1 cup raw cacao powder 2 tablespoons carob powder A handful of goji berries

Directions:

Prepare the crust, and for this, place all its ingredients in a food processor and pulse for 3 to 5 minutes until the thick paste comes together. Take a tart pan, pour crust mixture in it and spread and press the mixture evenly in the bottom and sides, and freeze until required. Prepare the filling, and for this, place all its ingredients in a food processor and pulse for 3 minutes until smooth. Pour the filling into the prepared tart, smooth the top and freeze for 3 hours until set. Cut tart into slices and then serve.

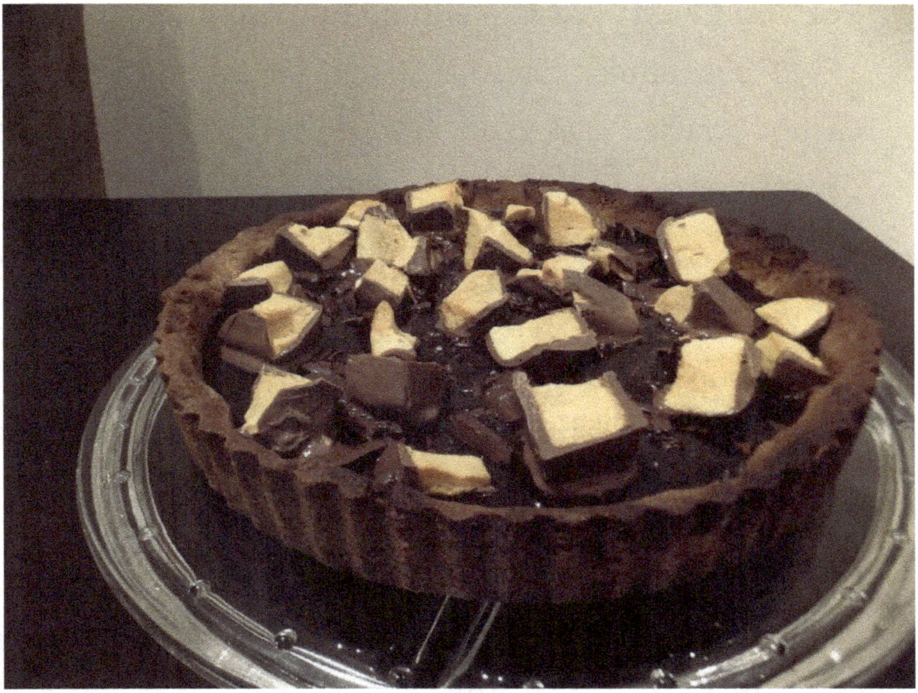

Chocolate Espresso Pie

Preparation time:3 hours and20 minutes Cooking time:0 minuteServings: 12

Ingredients:

For the Crust: 1/2 cup shredded coconut, unsweetened 1 1/2 cup dates, pitted 1/2 cup almonds 2 teaspoons cacao powder 1/4 cup maple syrup 3 tablespoons coconut oil

For the Filling: 3 dates, pitted 1 1/2 cup soaked cashews 1 tablespoon and 1 teaspoon espresso beans 3 tablespoons maple syrup 1 tablespoon and 1 teaspoon cacao powder 1/4 cup brewed coffee 1/2 cup cold water

Directions:

Prepare the crust, and for this, place all its ingredients in a food processor and pulse for 3 to 5 minutes until the thick paste comes together. Take an 8-inch cake pan, grease it with oil, pour crust mixture in it and spread and press the mixture evenly in the bottom and freeze until required. Prepare the filling, and for this, place cashews in a food processor, pour in water, and pulse for 2 minutes until smooth. Add dates, maple syrup, espresso beans, cocoa, and coffee, and blend until just mixed. Pour the filling into prepared pan, smooth the top and freeze for 3 hours until set. Cut pie into slices and then serve.

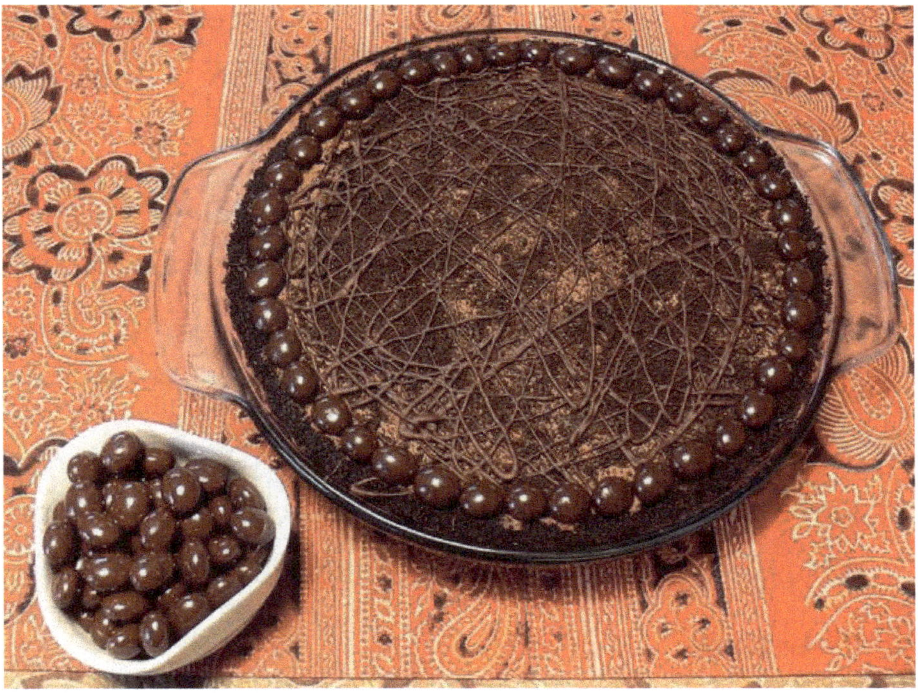

Peanut Butter Cheesecake

Preparation time: 5 minutes Cooking time: 15 minutes Servings: 8

Ingredients:

For the Crust:

1 cup dates, pitted, soaked in warm water for 10 minutes in water, drained 1/4 cup cocoa powder 3 Tablespoons melted coconut oil 1 cup rolled oats

For the Filling: 1 banana 1 1/2 cup cashews, soaked, drained 1/2 cup dates, pitted, soaked, drained 1/4 cup coconut oil 1 teaspoon vanilla extract, unsweetened 1/4 cup agave 1 cup peanut butter 1/2 cup coconut milk, chilled 1 tablespoon almond milk

For Garnish 2 tablespoons chocolate chips 2 tablespoons shredded coconut, unsweetened

Directions:

Prepare the crust, and for this, place all its ingredients in a food processor and pulse for 3 to 5 minutes until the thick paste comes together. Take a pie pan, grease it with oil, pour crust mixture in it and spread and press the mixture evenly in the bottom and along the sides, and freeze until required. Prepare the filling and for this, place all its ingredients in a food processor, and pulse for 2 minutes until smooth. Pour the filling into prepared pan, smooth the top, sprinkle chocolate chips and coconut on top and freeze for 4 hours until set. Cut cake into slices and then serve.

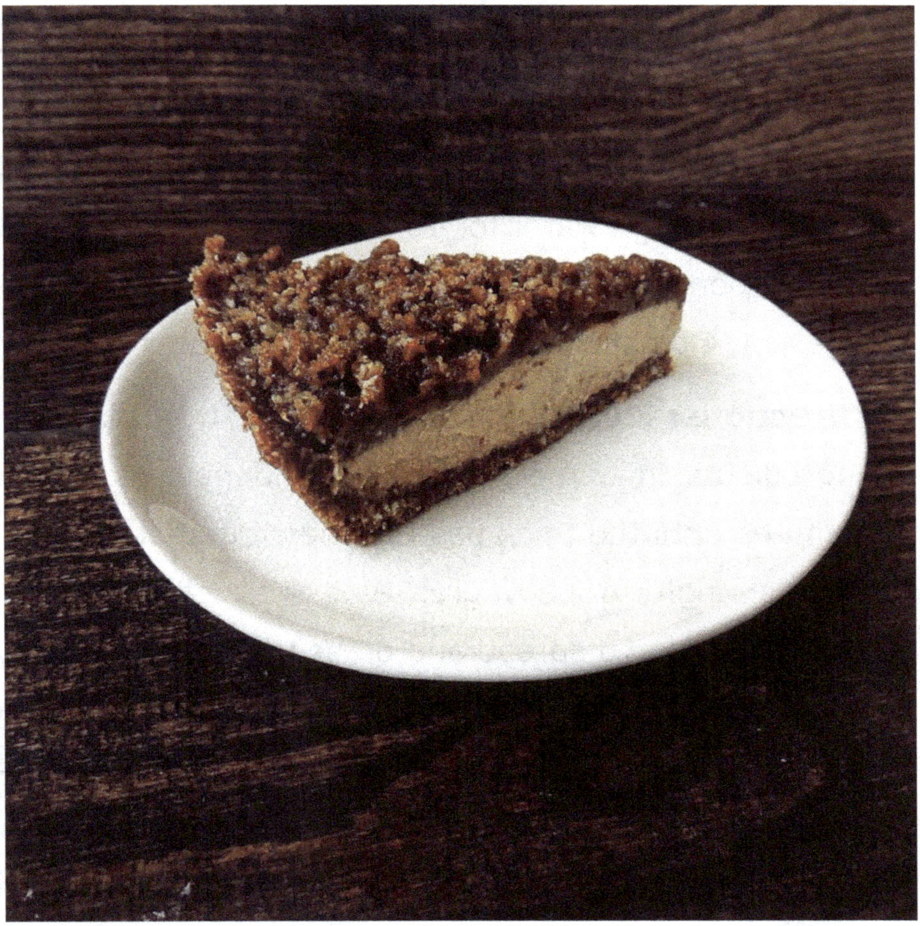

Chocolate Mint Grasshopper Pie

Preparation time:4 hours and 15 minutes Cooking time:0 minute Servings: 4

Ingredients:

For the Crust: 1 cup dates, soaked in warm water for 10 minutes in water, drained 1/8 teaspoons salt 1/2 cup pecans 1 teaspoons cinnamon 1/2 cup walnuts

For the Filling: ½ cup mint leaves 2 cups of cashews, soaked in warm water for 10 minutes in water, drained 2 tablespoons coconut oil 1/4 cup and 2 tablespoons of agave 1/4 teaspoons spirulina 1/4 cup water

Directions: Prepare the crust, and for this, place all its ingredients in a food processor and pulse for 3 to 5 minutes until the thick paste comes together. Take a 6-inch springform pan, grease it with oil, place crust mixture in it and spread and press the mixture evenly in the bottom and along the sides, and freeze until required. Prepare the filling and for this, place all its ingredients in a food processor, and pulse for 2 minutes until smooth. Pour the filling into prepared pan, smooth the top, and freeze for 4 hours until set. Cut pie into slices and then serve.

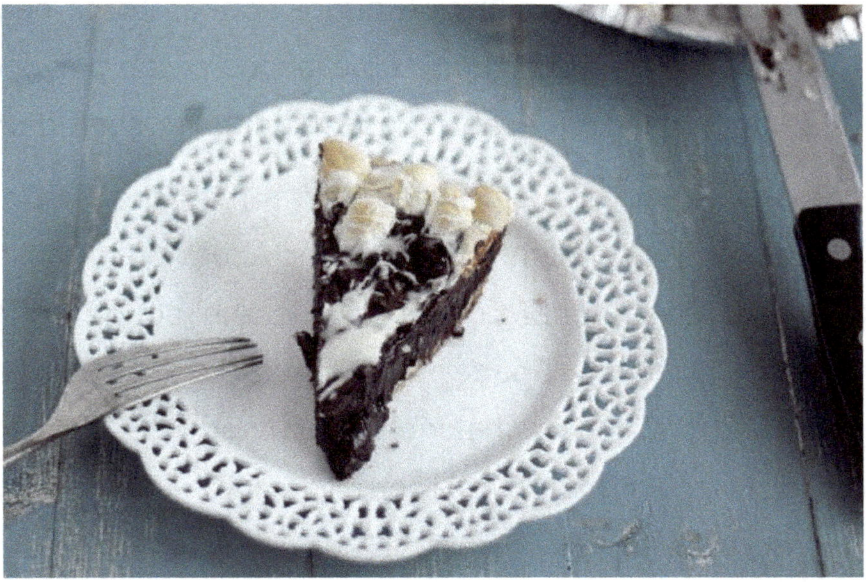

Black Bean Brownie Pops

Preparation time: 45 minutes Cooking time: 2 minutes Servings: 12

Ingredients:

3/4 cup chocolate chips 15 ounce cooked black beans 1 tablespoon maple syrup 5 tablespoons cacao powder 1/8 teaspoon sea salt 2 tablespoons sunflower seed butter

Directions: Place black beans in a food processor, add remaining ingredients, except for chocolate, and pulse for 2 minutes until combined and the dough starts to come together. Shape the dough into twelve balls, arrange them on a baking sheet lined with parchment paper, then insert a toothpick into each ball and refrigerate for 20 minutes. Then meat chocolate in the microwave for 2 minutes, and dip brownie pops in it until covered. Return the pops into the refrigerator for 10 minutes until set and then serve

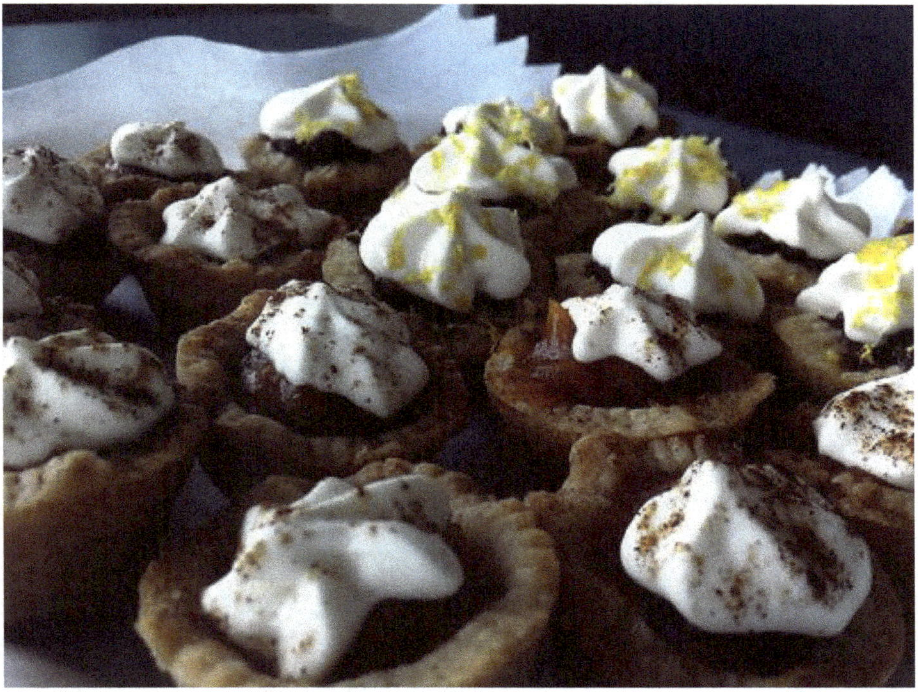

Peppermint Oreos

Preparation time: 2 hours Cooking time: 0 minute Servings: 12

Ingredients:

For the Cookies: 1 cup dates 2/3 cup brazil nuts 3 tablespoons carob powder 2/3 cup almonds 1/8 teaspoon sea salt 3 tablespoons water

For the Crème: 2 tablespoons almond butter 1 cup coconut chips 2 tablespoons melted coconut oil 1 cup coconut shreds 3 drops of peppermint oil 1/2 teaspoon vanilla powder

For the Dark Chocolate: 3/4 cup cacao powder 1/2 cup date paste 1/3 cup coconut oil, melted

Directions: Prepare the cookies, and for this, place all its ingredients in a food processor and pulse for 3 to 5 minutes until the dough comes together. Then place the dough between two parchment sheets, roll the dough, then cut out twenty-four cookies of the desired shape and freeze until solid. Prepare the crème, and for this, place all its ingredients in a food processor and pulse for 2 minutes until smooth. When cookies have harden, sandwich crème in between the cookies by placing dollops on top of a cookie and then pressing it with another cookie. Freeze the cookies for 30 minutes and in the meantime, prepare chocolate and for this, place all its ingredients in a bowl and whisk until combined. Dip frouncesen cookie sandwich into chocolate, at least two times, and then freeze for another 30 minutes until chocolate has hardened. Serve straight away.

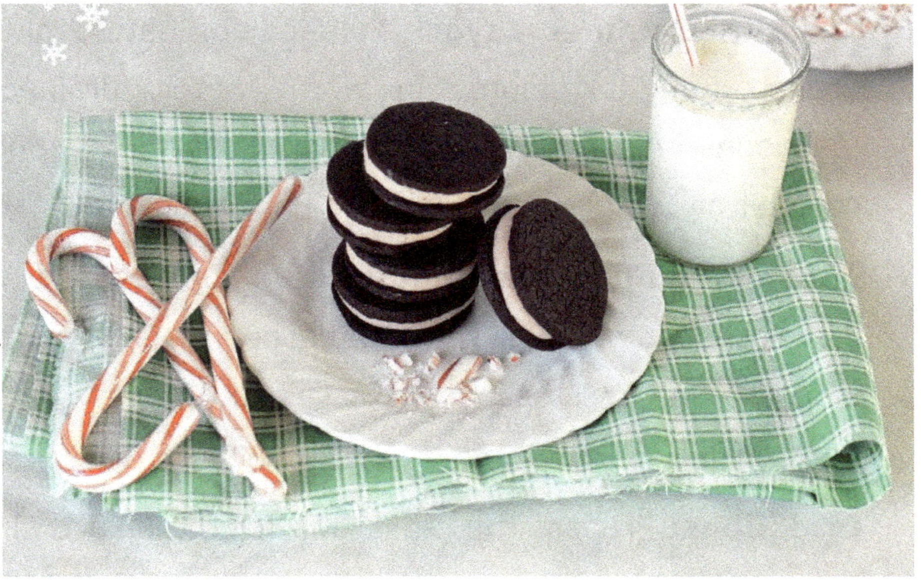

Snickers Pie

Preparation time: 4 hours Cooking time: 0 minute Servings: 16

Ingredients:

For the Crust: 12 Medjool dates, pitted 1 cup dried coconut, unsweetened 5 tablespoons cocoa powder 1/2 teaspoon sea salt 1 teaspoon vanilla extract, unsweetened 1 cup almonds

For the Caramel Layer: 10 Medjool dates, pitted, soaked for 10 minutes in warm water, drained 2 teaspoons vanilla extract, unsweetened 3 teaspoons coconut oil 3 tablespoons almond butter, unsalted

For the Peanut Butter Mousse: 3/4 cup peanut butter 2 tablespoons maple syrup 1/2 teaspoon vanilla extract, unsweetened 1/8 teaspoon sea salt 28 ounces coconut milk, chilled

Directions: Prepare the crust, and for this, place all its ingredients in a food processor and pulse for 3 to 5 minutes until the thick paste comes together. Take a baking pan, line it with parchment paper, place crust mixture in it and spread and press the mixture evenly in the bottom, and freeze until required. Prepare the caramel layer, and for this, place all its ingredients in a food processor and pulse for 2 minutes until smooth. Pour the caramel on top of the prepared crust, smooth the top and freeze for 30 minutes until set. Prepare the mousse and for this, separate coconut milk and its solid, then add solid from coconut milk into a food processor, add remaining ingredients and then pulse for 1 minute until smooth. Top prepared mousse over caramel layer, and then freeze for 3 hours until set. Serve straight away.

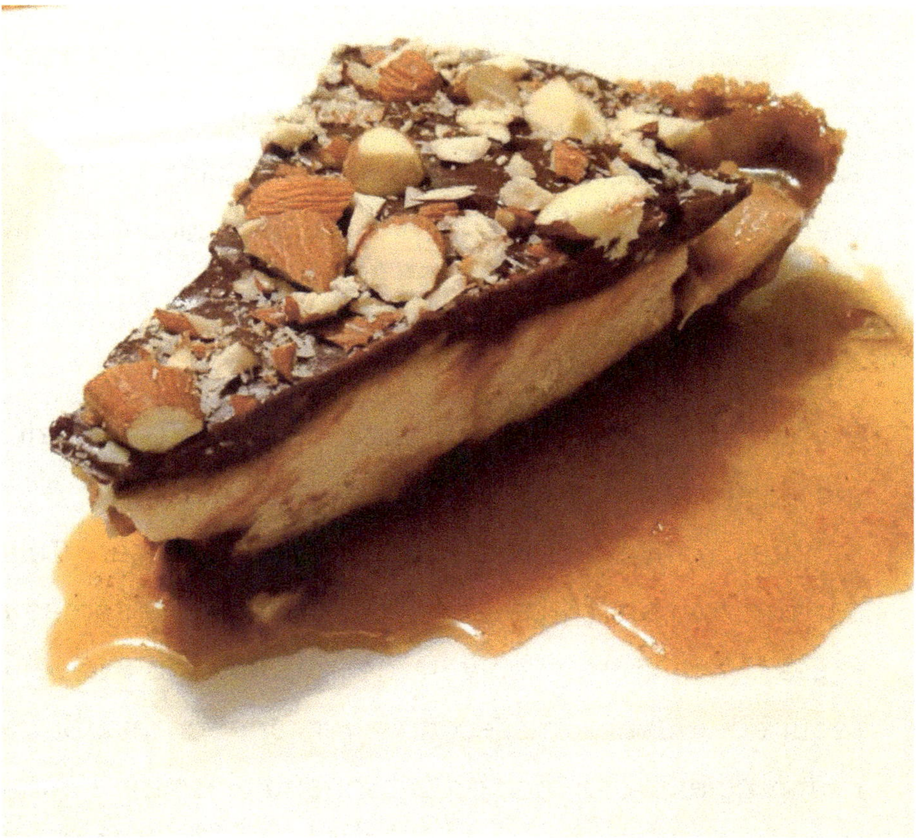

Coconut Ice Cream Cheesecake

Preparation time: 3 hours Cooking time: 0 minute Servings: 4

Ingredients:

For the First Layer: 1 cup mixed nuts 3/4 cup dates, soaked for 10 minutes in warm water 2 tablespoons almond milk

For the Second Layer: 1 medium avocado, diced 1 cup cashew nuts, soaked for 10 minutes in warm water 3 cups strawberries, sliced 1 tablespoon chia seeds, soaked in 3 tablespoons soy milk 1/2 cup agave 1 cup melted coconut oil 1/2 cup shredded coconut 1 lime, juiced

Directions:

Prepare the first layer, and for this, place all its ingredients in a food processor and pulse for 3 to 5 minutes until the thick paste comes together. Take a springform pan, place crust mixture in it and spread and press the mixture evenly in the bottom, and freeze until required. Prepare the second layer, and for this, place all its ingredients in a food processor and pulse for 2 minutes until smooth. Pour the second layer on top of the first layer, smooth the top, and freeze for 4 hours until hard. Serve straight away.

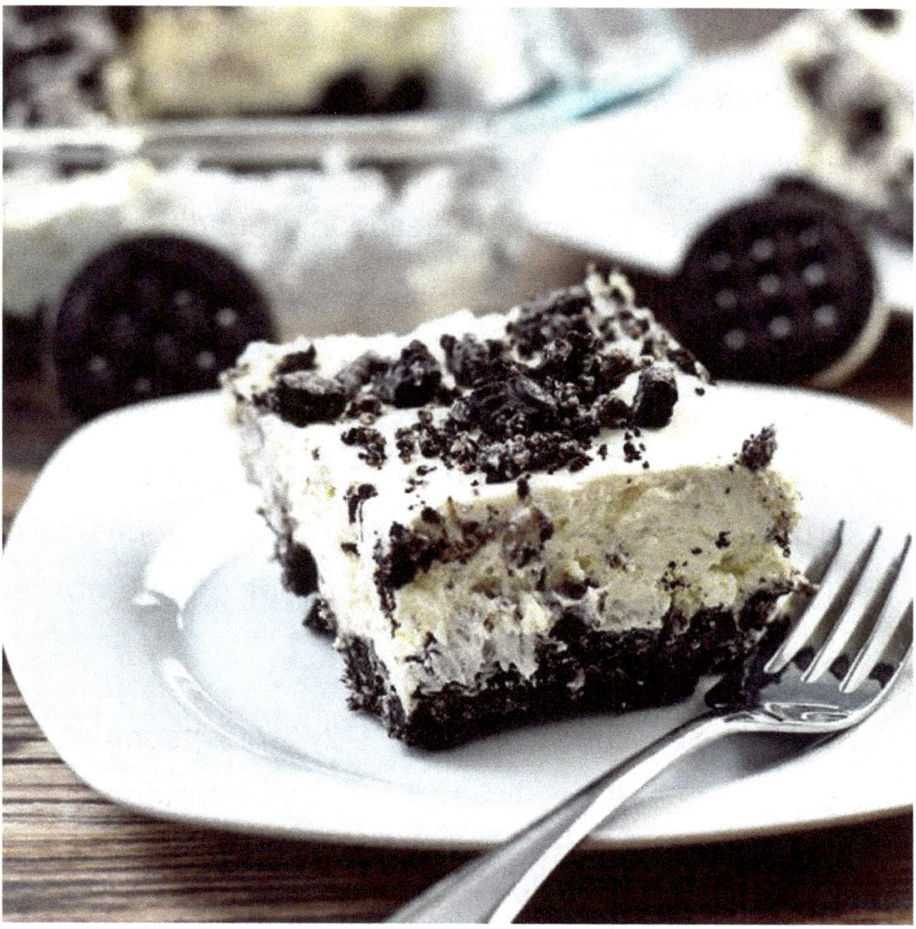

Chocolate Peanut Butter Cake

Preparation time: 5 minutes Cooking time: 0 minute Servings: 8

Ingredients:

For the Base: 1 tablespoon ground flaxseeds 1/8 cup millet 3/4 cup peanuts 1/4 cup and 2 tablespoons shredded coconut unsweetened 1 teaspoon hemp oil 1/2 cup flake oats

For the Date Layer: 1 tablespoon ground flaxseed 1 cup dates 1 tablespoon hemp hearts 2 tablespoons coconut 3 tablespoons cacao

For the Chocolate Layer: 3/4 cup coconut flour 2 tablespoons and 2 teaspoons cacao 1 tablespoon maple syrup 8 tablespoons warm water 2 tablespoons coconut oil 1/2 cup coconut milk 2 tablespoons ground flaxseed

For the Chocolate Topping:

7 ounces coconut cream 2 1/2 tablespoons cacao 1 teaspoon agave For Assembly: 1/2 cup almond butter

Directions:

Prepare the crust, and for this, place all its ingredients in a food processor and pulse for 3 to 5 minutes until the thick paste comes together. Take a loaf tin, grease it with oil, place crust mixture in it and spread and press the mixture evenly in the bottom and along the sides, and freeze until required. Prepare the date layer, and for this, place all its ingredients in a food processor and pulse for 2 minutes until smooth. Prepare the chocolate layer, and for this, place flour and flax in a bowl and stir until combined. Take a saucepan, add remaining ingredients, stir until mixed and cook for 5 minutes until melted and smooth. Add it into the flour mixture, stir until dough comes together, and set aside. Prepare the chocolate topping, place all its ingredients in a food processor and pulse for 3 to 5 minutes until smooth. Press date layer into the base layer, refrigerate for 1 hour, then press chocolate layer on its top, finish with chocolate topping, refrigerate for 3 hours and serve.

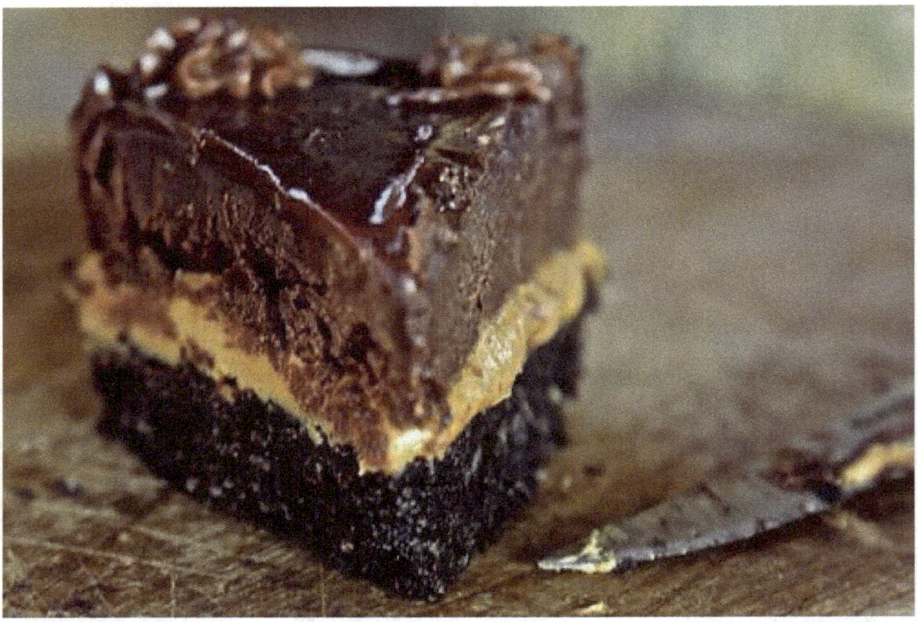

Brownie Batter

Preparation time: 5 minutes Cooking time: 0 minute Servings: 4

Ingredients:

4 Medjool dates, pitted, soaked in warm water 1.5 ounces chocolate, unsweetened, melted 2 tablespoons maple syrup 4 tablespoons tahini ½ teaspoon vanilla extract, unsweetened 1 tablespoon cocoa powder, unsweetened 1/8 teaspoon sea salt 1/8 teaspoon espresso powder 2 to 4 tablespoons almond milk, unsweetened

Directions:

Place all the ingredients in a food processor and process for 2 minutes until combined. Set aside until required

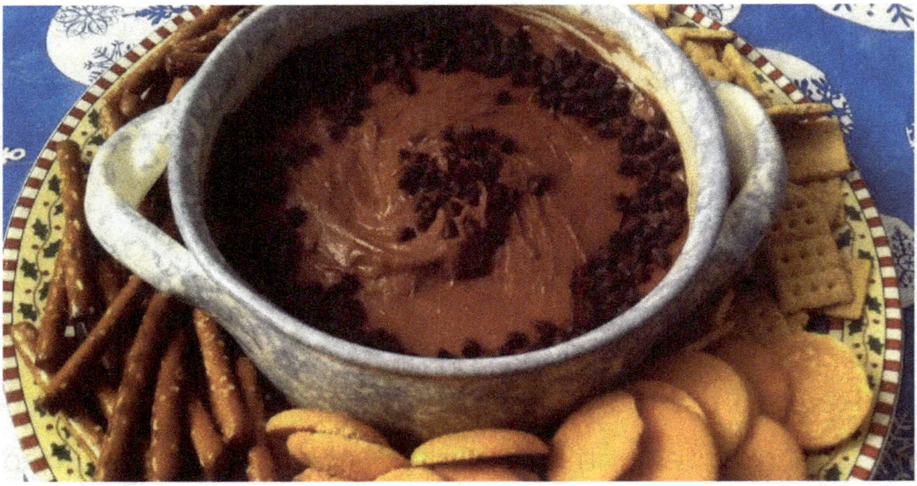

Blueberry Mousse

Preparation time: 20 minutes Cooking time: 0 minute Servings: 2

Ingredients:

1 cup wild blueberries 1 cup cashews, soaked for 10 minutes, drained 1/2 teaspoon berry powder 2 tablespoons coconut oil, melted 1 tablespoon lemon juice 1 teaspoon vanilla extract, unsweetened 1/4 cup hot water

Directions:

Place all the ingredients in a food processor and process for 2 minutes until smooth. Set aside until required.

Homemade Basics, Sauces, and Condiments

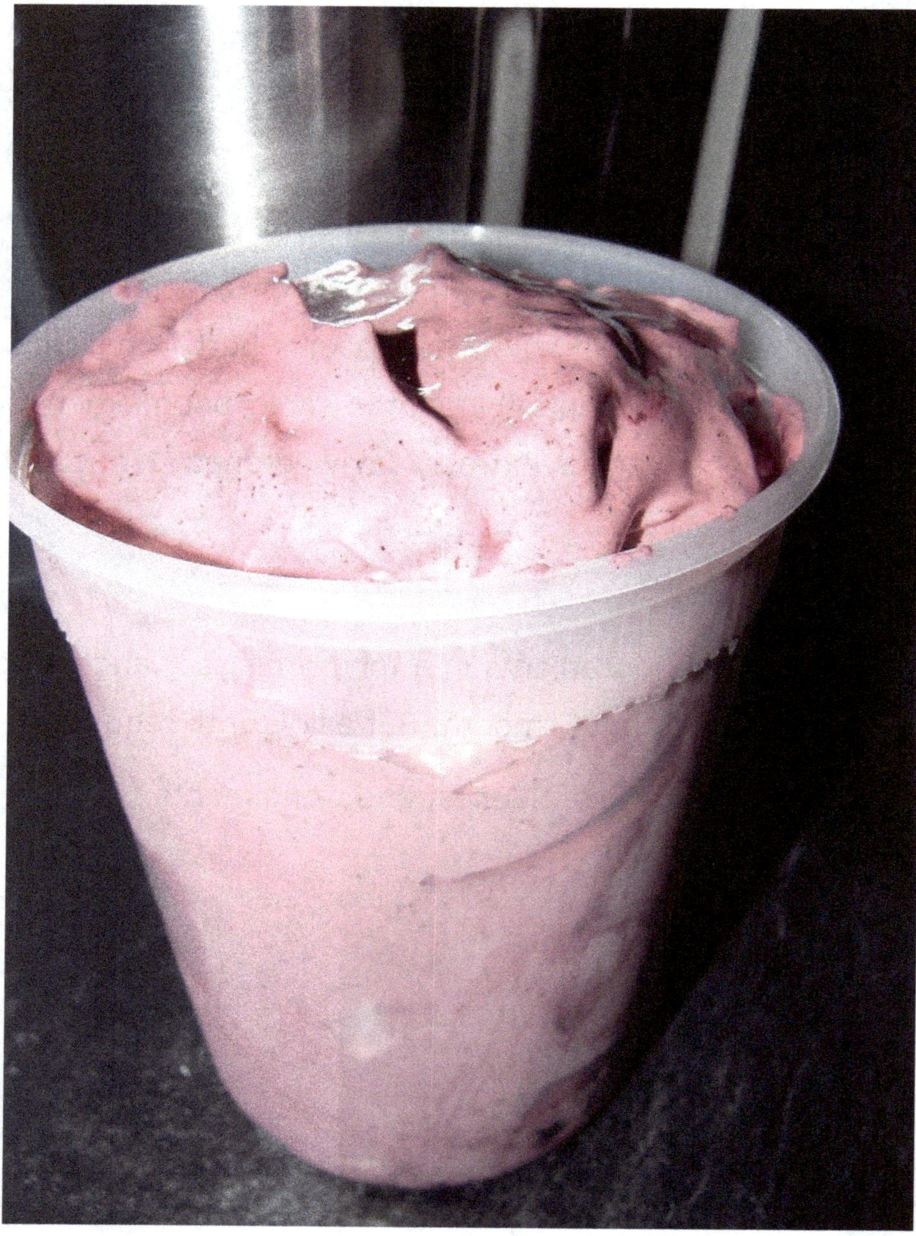

Garlic, Parmesan and White Bean Hummus

Preparation time: 5 minutes Cooking time: 0 minute Servings: 6

Ingredients:

4 cloves of garlic, peeled 12 ounces cooked white beans 1/8 teaspoon salt ½ lemon, zested 1 tablespoon lemon juice 1 tablespoon olive oil 3 tablespoon water 1/4 cup grated Parmesan cheese

Directions:

Place all the ingredients in the order in a food processor or blender and then pulse for 3 to 5 minutes at high speed until the thick mixture comes together. Tip the hummus in a bowl and then serve.

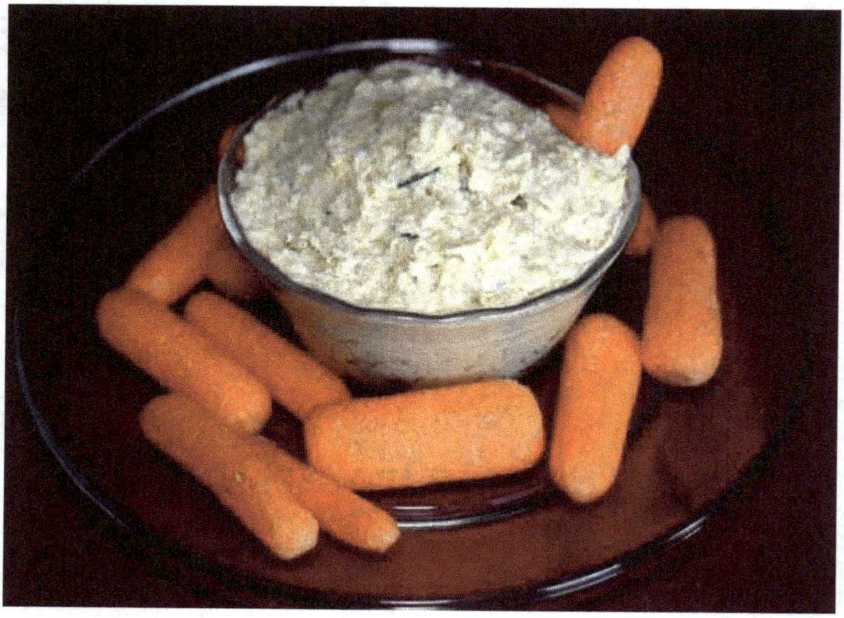

Kale and Walnut Pesto

Preparation time: 5 minutes Cooking time: 10 minutes Servings: 4

Ingredients:

1/2 bunch kale, leaves chop 1/2 cup chopped walnuts 2 cloves of garlic, peeled 1/4 cup nutritional yeast ½ of lemon, juiced 1/4 cup olive oil ¼ teaspoon. ground black pepper 1/3 teaspoon. salt

Directions:

Place a large pot filled with water over medium heat, bring it to boil, then add kale and boil for 5 minutes until tender. Drain kale, then transfer it in a blender, add remaining ingredients and then pulse for 5 minutes until smooth. Serve straight away.

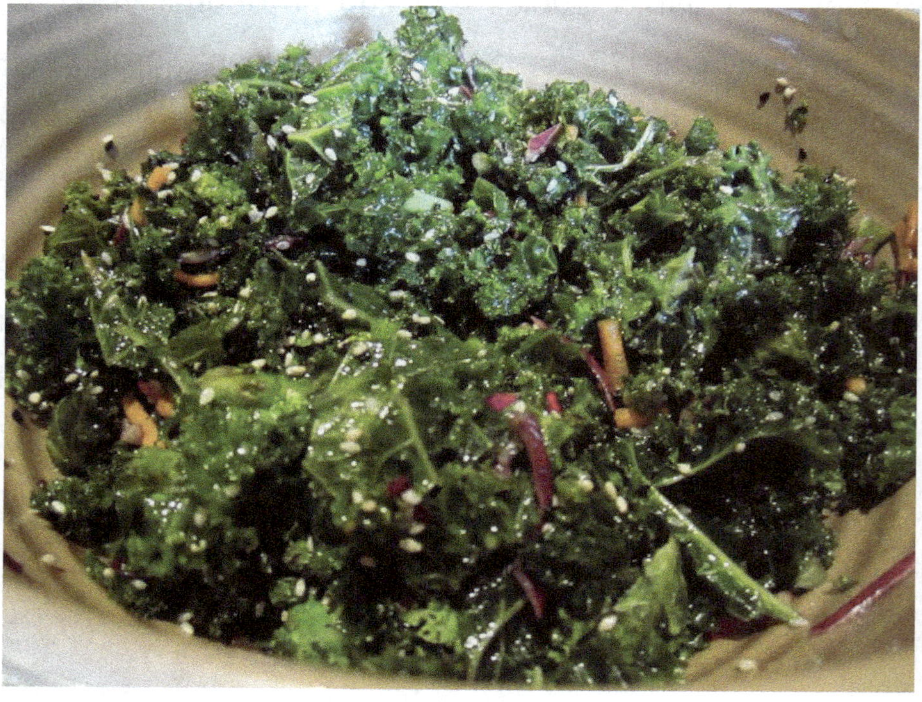

Barbecue Tahini Sauce

Preparation time: 5 minutes Cooking time: 0 minute Servings: 8

Ingredients:

6 tablespoons tahini 3/4 teaspoon garlic powder 1/8 teaspoon red chili powder 2 teaspoons maple syrup 1/4 teaspoon salt 3 teaspoons molasses 3 teaspoons apple cider vinegar 1/4 teaspoon liquid smoke 10 teaspoons tomato paste 1/2 cup water

Directions:

Place all the ingredients in the order in a food processor or blender and then pulse for 3 to 5 minutes at high speed until smooth. Tip the sauce in a bowl and then serve.

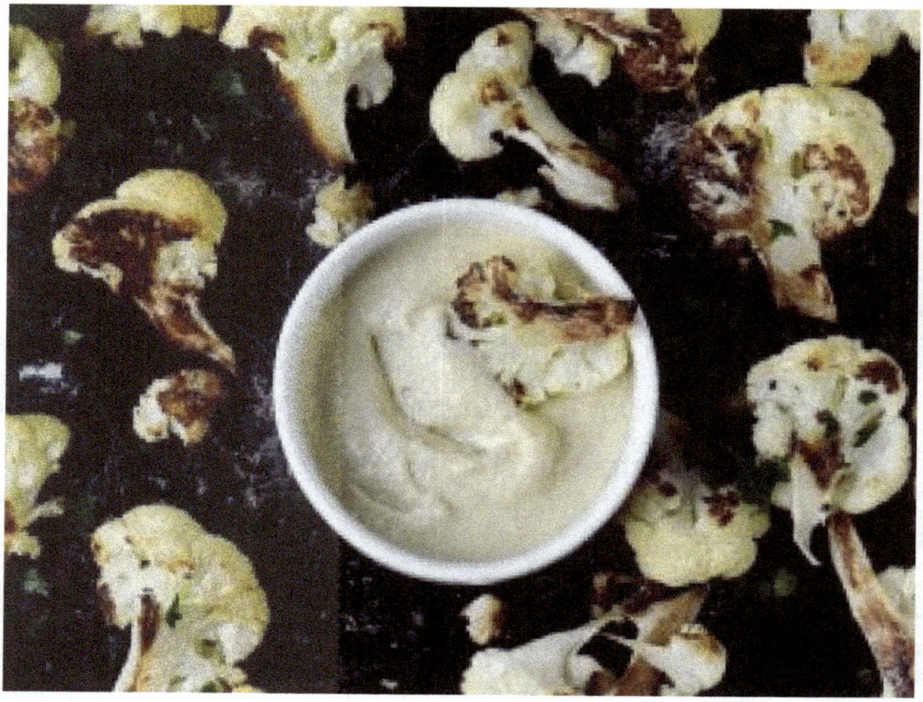

Cashew Yogurt

Preparation time:12 hours and 5 minutes Cooking time:0 minute Servings: 8

Ingredients:

3 probiotic supplements 2 2/3 cups cashews, unsalted , soaked in warm water for 15 minutes 1/4 teaspoon sea salt 4 tablespoon lemon juice 1 1/2 cup water

Directions:

Drain the cashews, add them into the food processor, then add remaining ingredients, except for probiotic supplements, and pulse for 2 minutes until smooth. Tip the mixture in a bowl, add probiotic supplements, stir until mixed, then cover the bowl with a cheesecloth and let it stand for 12 hours in a dark and cool room. Serve straight away.

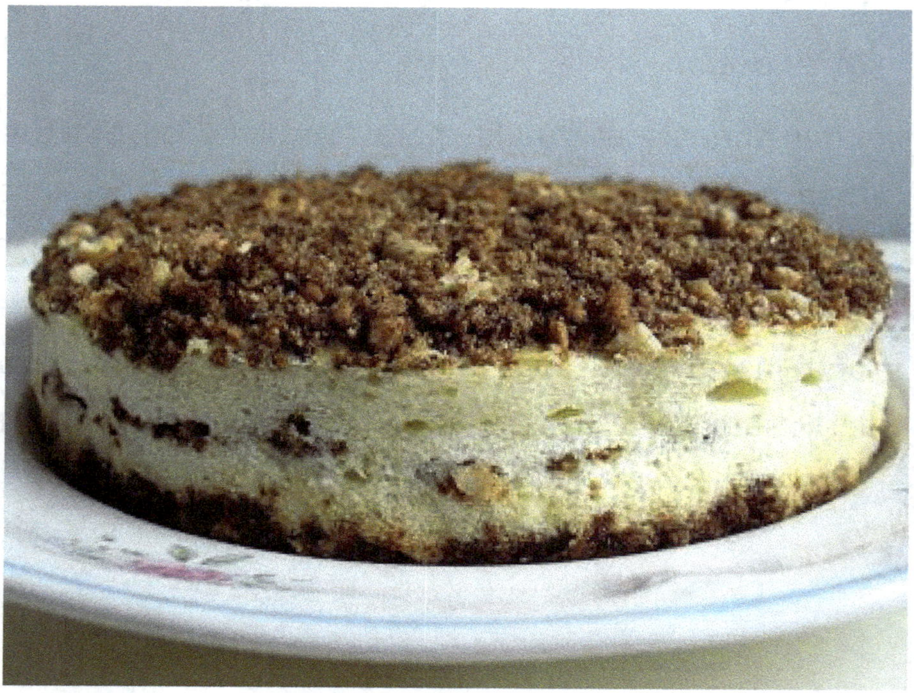

Thai Peanut Sauce

Preparation time: 10 minutes Cooking time: 10 minutes Servings: 4

Ingredients:

2 tablespoons ground peanut, and more for topping 2 tablespoons Thai red curry paste ½ teaspoon salt 1 tablespoon sugar 1/2 cup creamy peanut butter 2 tablespoons apple cider vinegar 3/4 cup coconut milk, unsweetened

Directions:

Take a saucepan, place it over low heat, add all the ingredients, whisk well until combined, and then bring the sauce to simmer. Then remove the pan from heat, top with ground peanuts, and serve.

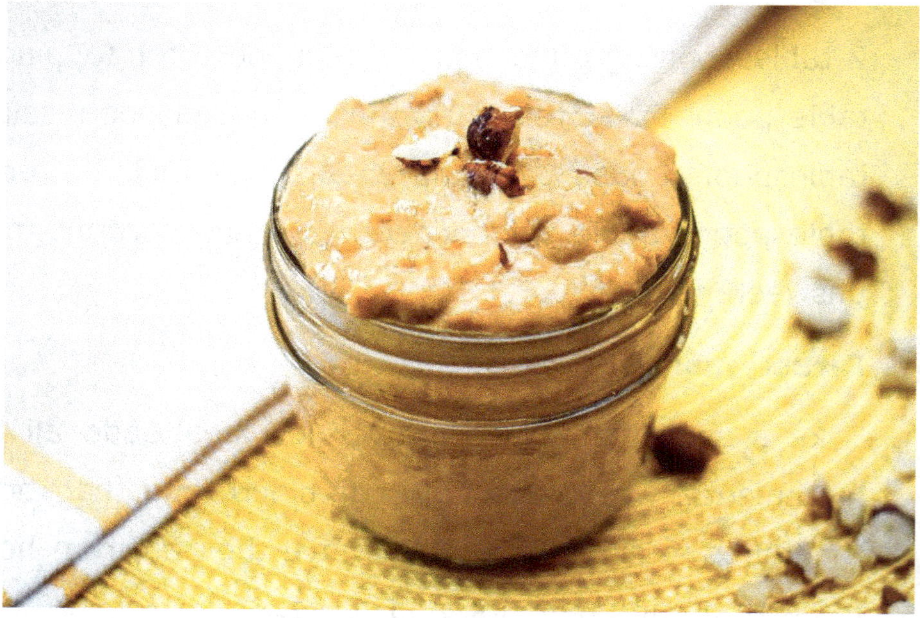

Spicy Red Wine Tomato Sauce

Preparation time: 5 minutes Cooking time: 1 hour Servings: 4

Ingredients:

28 ounces puree of whole tomatoes, peeled 4 cloves of garlic, peeled 1 tablespoon dried basil ¼ teaspoon ground black pepper 1 tablespoon dried oregano ¼ teaspoon red pepper flakes 1 tablespoon dried sage 1 tablespoon dried thyme 3 teaspoon coconut sugar 1/2 of lemon, juice 1/4 cup red wine

Directions:

Take a large saucepan, place it over medium heat, add tomatoes and remaining ingredients, stir and simmer for 1 hour or more until thickened and cooked. Serve sauce over pasta.

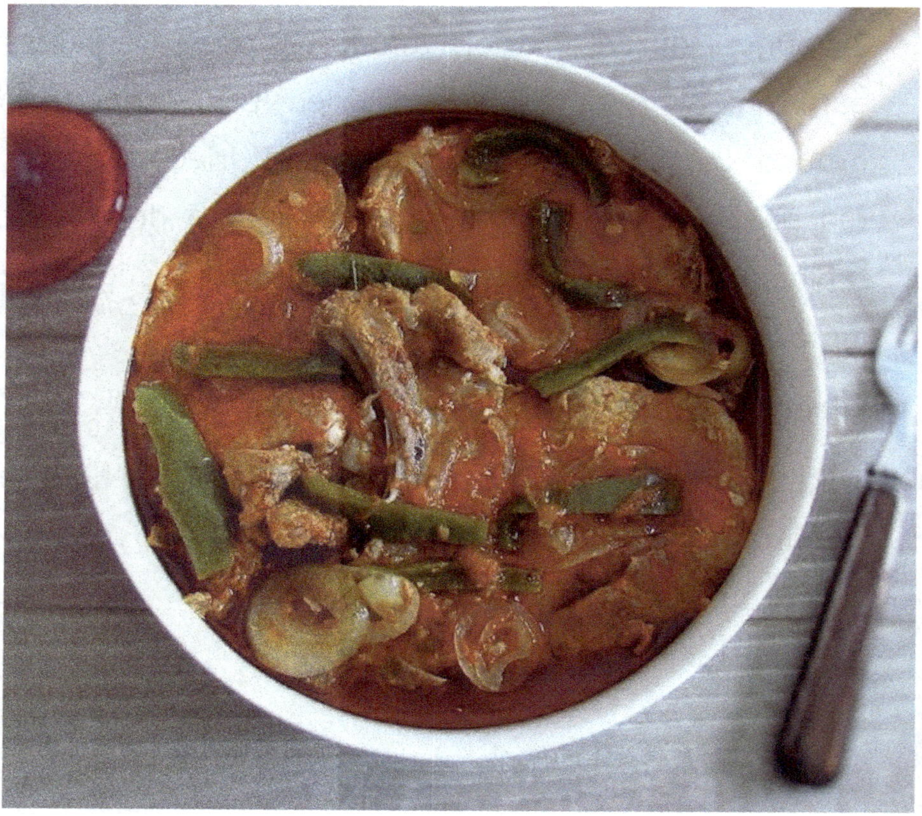

Strawberry-Chocolate Yogurt Shake

Preparation time: 5 minutes Cooking time: 0 minutes Servings: 1

Ingredients:

½ cup whole milk yogurt 4 strawberries, chopped 1 tbsp cocoa powder 3 tbsp coconut oil 1 tbsp pepitas What you'll need from the store cupboard: 1 ½ cups water 1 packet Stevia, or more to taste

Directions

Add all ingredients in a blender. Blend until smooth and creamy. Serve and enjoy.

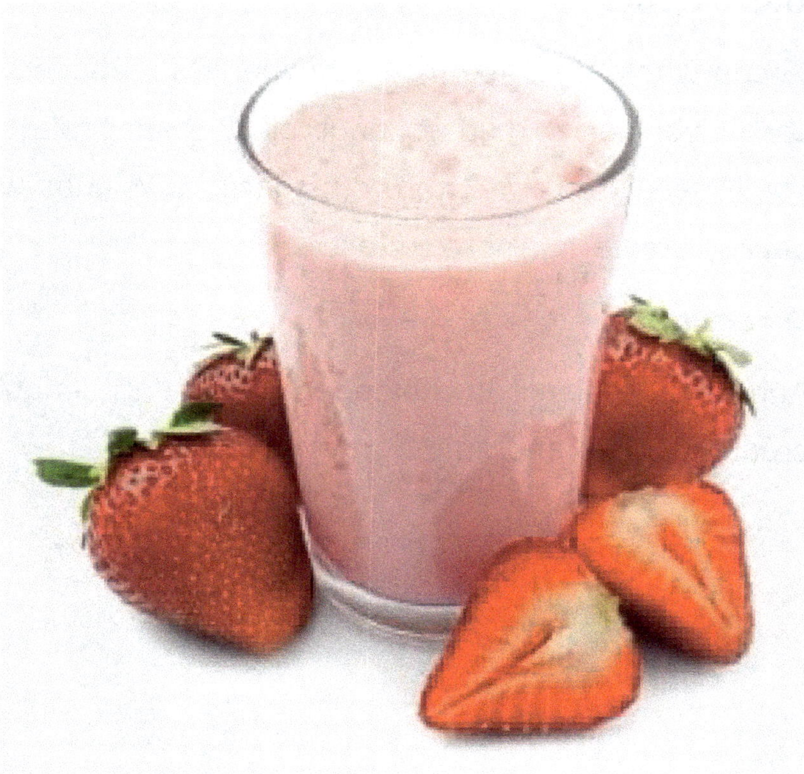

Berry-Choco Goodness Shake

Preparation time: 5 minutes Cooking time: 0 minutes Servings: 1

Ingredients:

½ cup half and half ¼ cup raspberries ¼ cup blackberry ¼ cup strawberries, chopped 3 tbsps avocado oil What you'll need from the store cupboard: 1 packet Stevia, or more to taste 1 tbsp cocoa powder 1 ½ cups water

Directions

Add all ingredients in a blender. Blend until smooth and creamy. Serve and enjoy

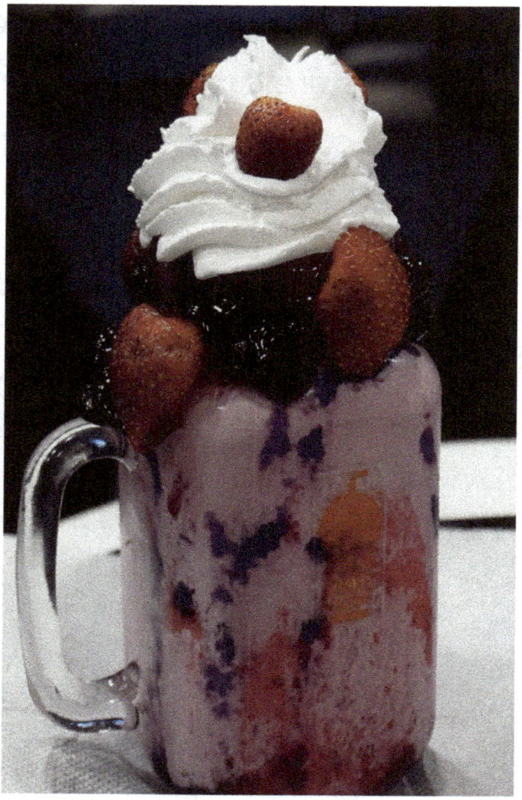

Strawberry-Coconut Shake

Preparation time: 5 minutes Cooking time: 0 minutes Servings: 1

Ingredients:

½ cup whole milk yogurt 3 tbsp MCT oil ¼ cup strawberries, chopped 1 tbsp coconut flakes, unsweetened 1 tbsp hemp seeds What you'll need from the store cupboard: 1 ½ cups water 1 packet Stevia, or more to taste

Directions

Add all ingredients in a blender. Blend until smooth and creamy. Serve and enjoy.

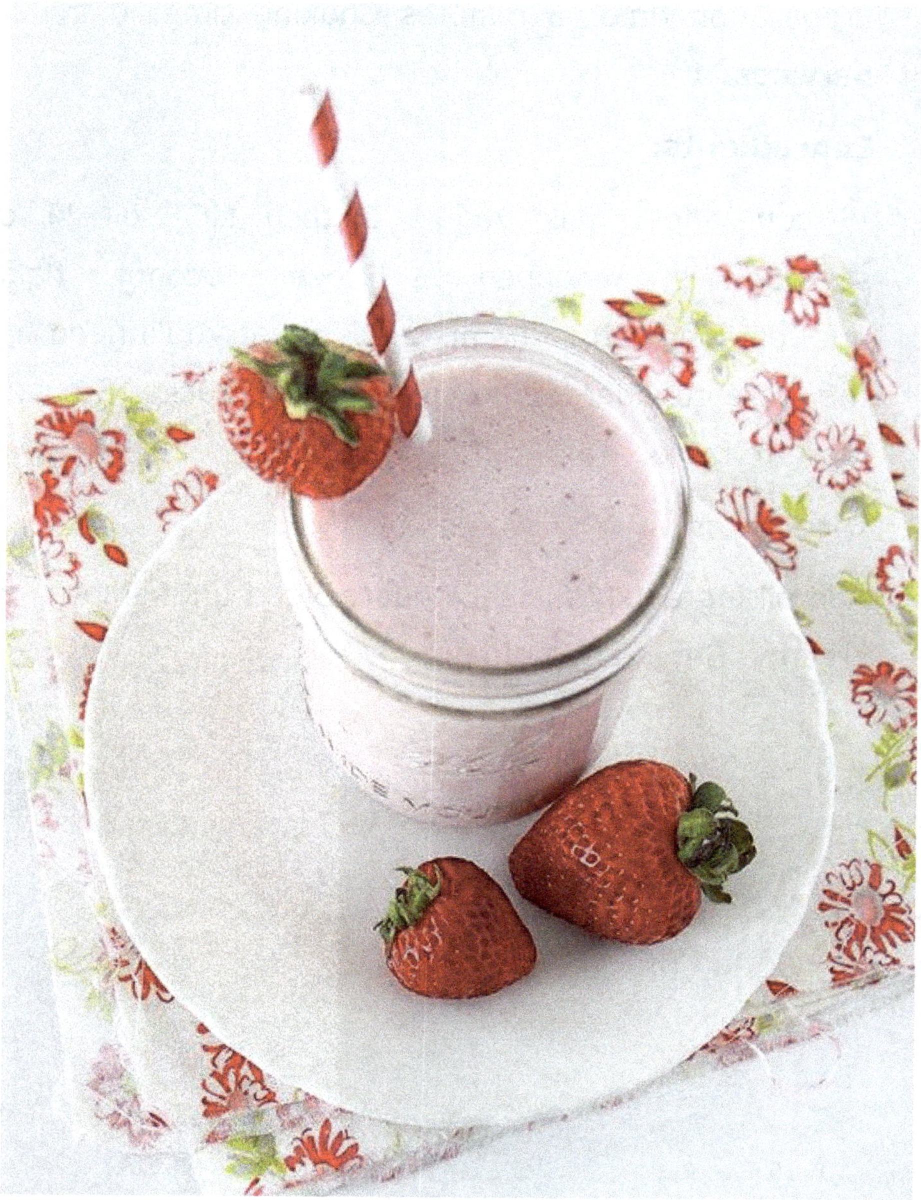

Blackberry-Chocolate Shake

Preparation time: 5 minutes Cooking time: 0 minutes Servings: 1

Ingredients:

½ cup half and half 1 tbsp blackberries 3 tbsps MCT oil 1 tbsp Dutch-processed cocoa powder 2 tbsp Macadamia nuts, chopped What you'll need from the store cupboard: 1 ½ cups water 1 packet Stevia, or more to taste

Directions

Add all ingredients in a blender. Blend until smooth and creamy. Serve and enjoy.

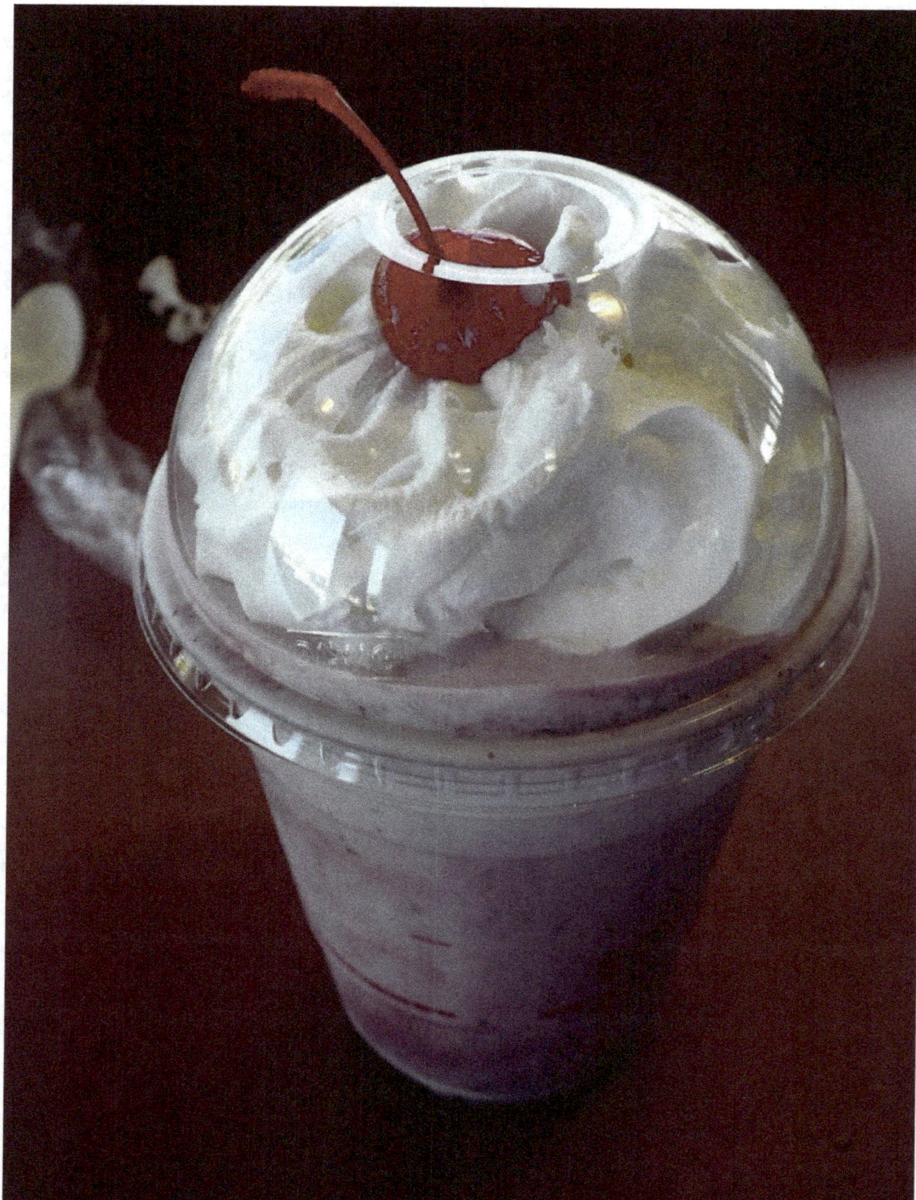

Italian Greens and Yogurt Shake

Preparation time: 5 minutes Cooking time: 0 minutes Servings: 1

Ingredients:

½ cup half and half ½ cup Italian greens 1 packet Stevia, or more to taste 1 tbsp hemp seeds What you'll need from the store cupboard: 3 tbsp coconut oil 1 cup water

Directions Add all ingredients in a blender. Blend until smooth and creamy. Serve and enjoy.

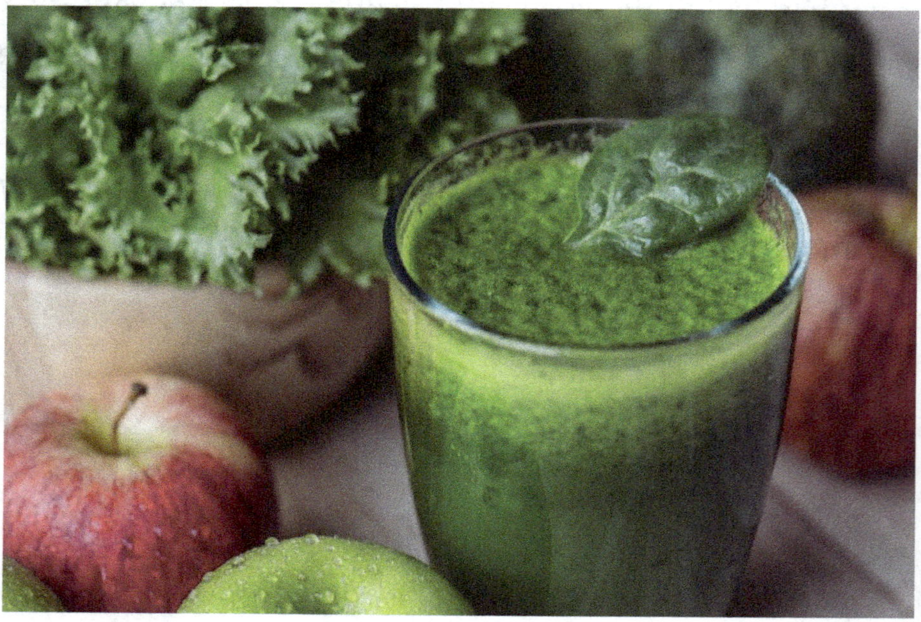

Hazelnut-Lettuce Yogurt Shake

Preparation time: 5 minutes Cooking time: 0 minutes Servings: 1

Ingredients:

1 cup whole milk yogurt 1 cup lettuce chopped 1 tbsp Hazelnut chopped What you'll need from the store cupboard: 1 packet Stevia, or more to taste 1 tbsp olive oil 1 cup water

Directions

Add all ingredients in a blender. Blend until smooth and creamy. Serve and enjoy.

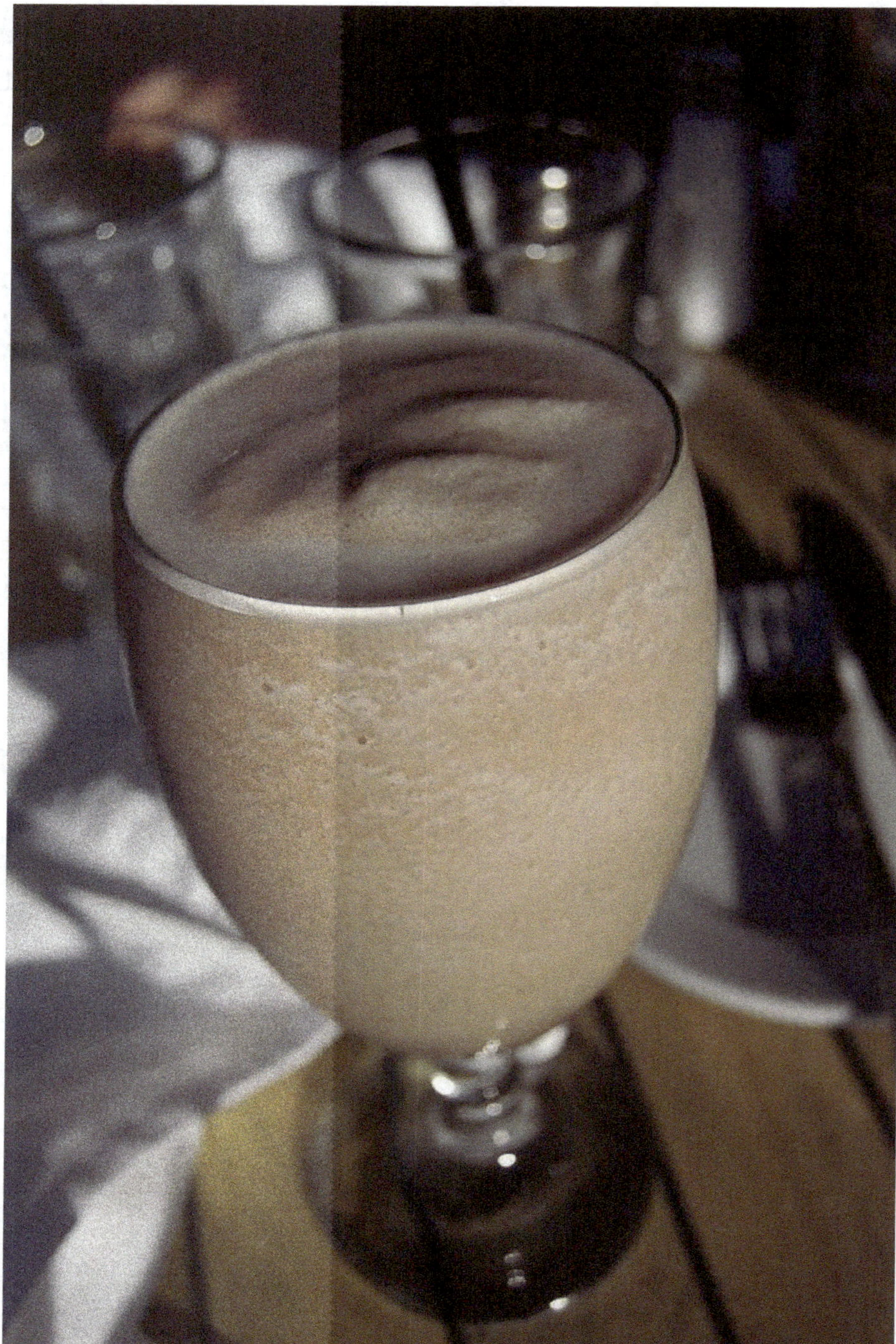

Baby Kale and Yogurt Smoothie

Preparation time: 5 minutes Cooking time: 0 minutes Servings: 1

Ingredients:

½ cup whole milk yogurt ½ cup baby kale greens 1 packet Stevia, or more to taste 3 tbsps MCT oil ½ tbsp sunflower seeds What you'll need from the store cupboard: 1 cup water

Directions

Add all ingredients in a blender. Blend until smooth and creamy. Serve and enjoy.

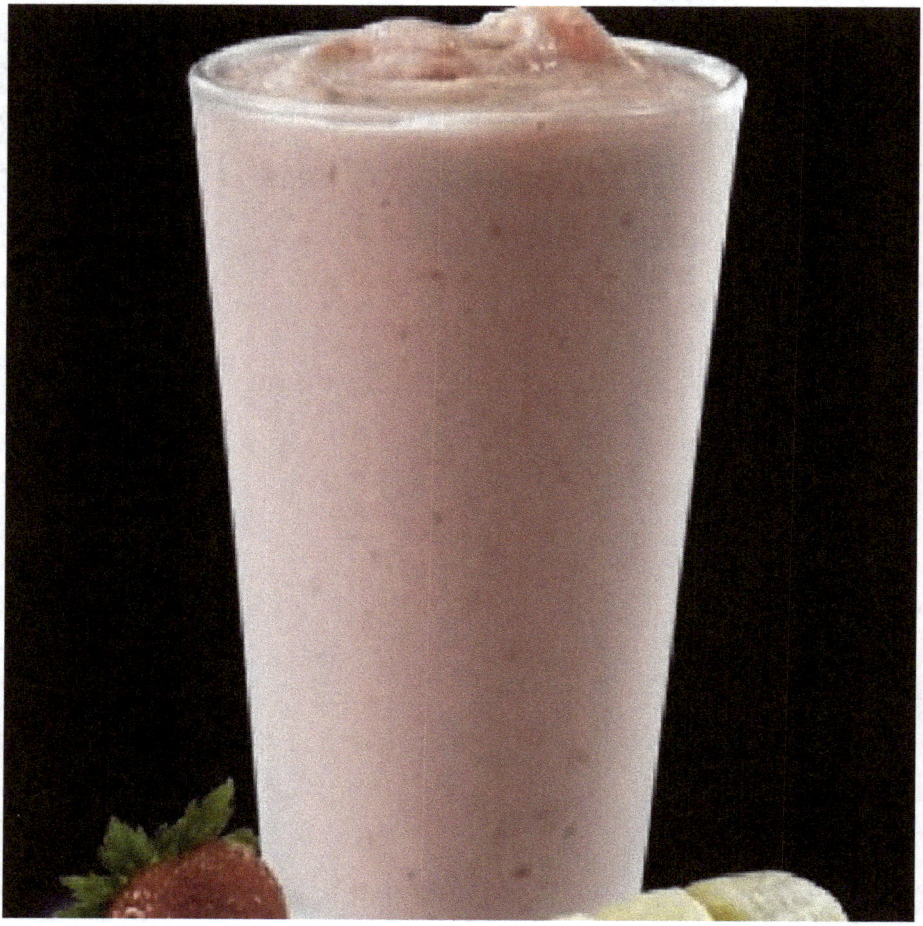

Fudgy Almond Bars

Servings:8 Preparation Time: 10 Minutes

Ingredients:

1 cup almond flour 1 ounce dark chocolate or sugar-free chocolate chips 1/2 cup almond butter 1/2 cup unsalted butter (melted and divided) 1/2 teaspoon ground cinnamon 1/2 teaspoon vanilla extract 1/4 cup heavy cream 1/8 teaspoon xanthan gum 6 tablespoons powdered erythritol (divided)

Directions

for Cooking: Line a 9x10-inch baking dish and preheat oven to 400oF. In a medium mixing bowl, whisk well cinnamon, 2 tbsp powdered erythritol, ¼ cup melted butter, and almond flour. Evenly spread mixture on bottom of prepared pan and pop in the oven. Bake until golden brown, around 10 minutes. Once done, remove from oven and cool completely. In another mixing bowl, beat well 4 tbsp powdered erythritol, remaining butter, almond butter, and heavy cream. Stir in xanthan gum and vanilla. Mix well. Evenly spread mixture on top of cooled crust. Sprinkle choco chips and refrigerate overnight. Evenly slice into 8 bars and enjoy.

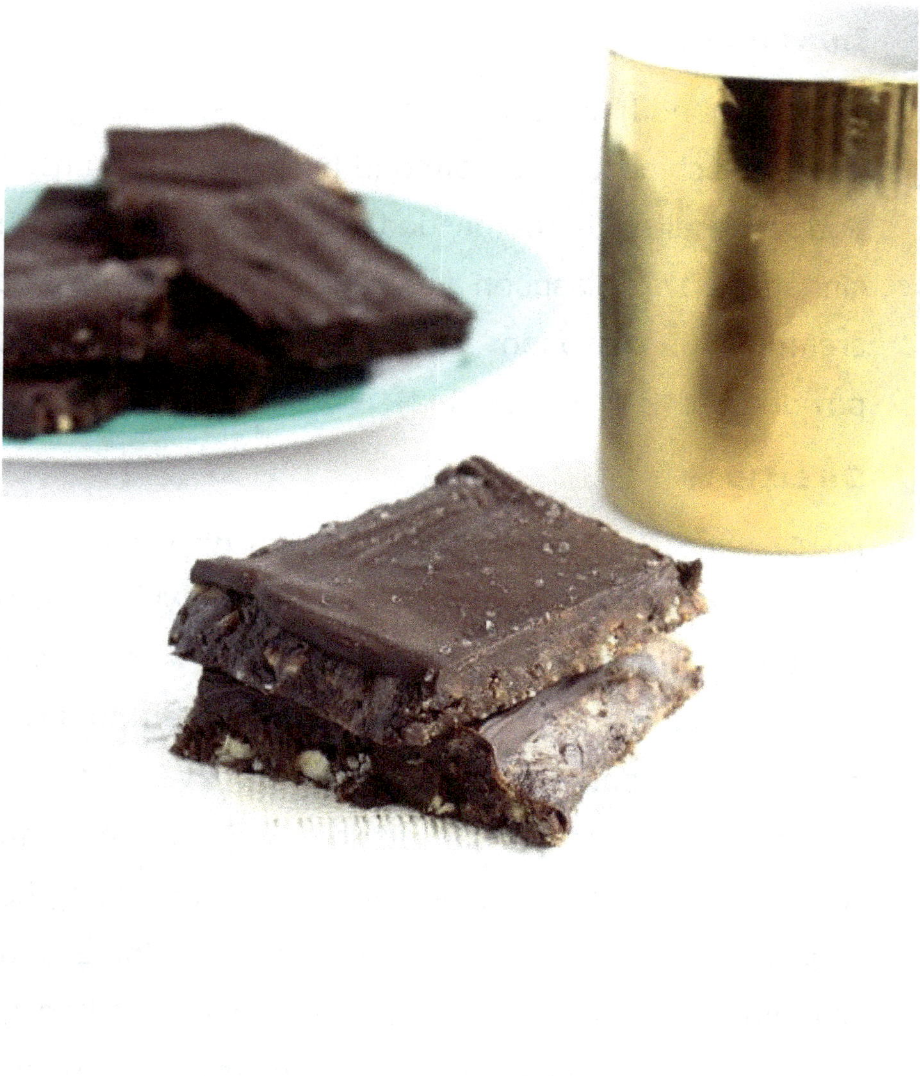

Banana Pudding Approved

Servings:1 Preparation Time: 5 Minutes

Ingredients:

1 large egg yolk 1/2 cup heavy cream 1/2 tsp banana extract 1/2 tsp xanthan gum 3 tbsp powdered erythritol

Directions

for Cooking: Place a large saucepan with 1-inch of water on medium high fire. Place a small pot inside the saucepan. Add powdered erythritol, egg yolk, and heavy cream in small pot. Whisk well to mix and continue whisking until thickened. Stir in xanthan gum and continue whisking to mix and thicken more. Add salt and banana extract. Mix well. Transfer to a small bowl and cover top completely with cling wrap. Refrigerate for 4 hours and enjoy.

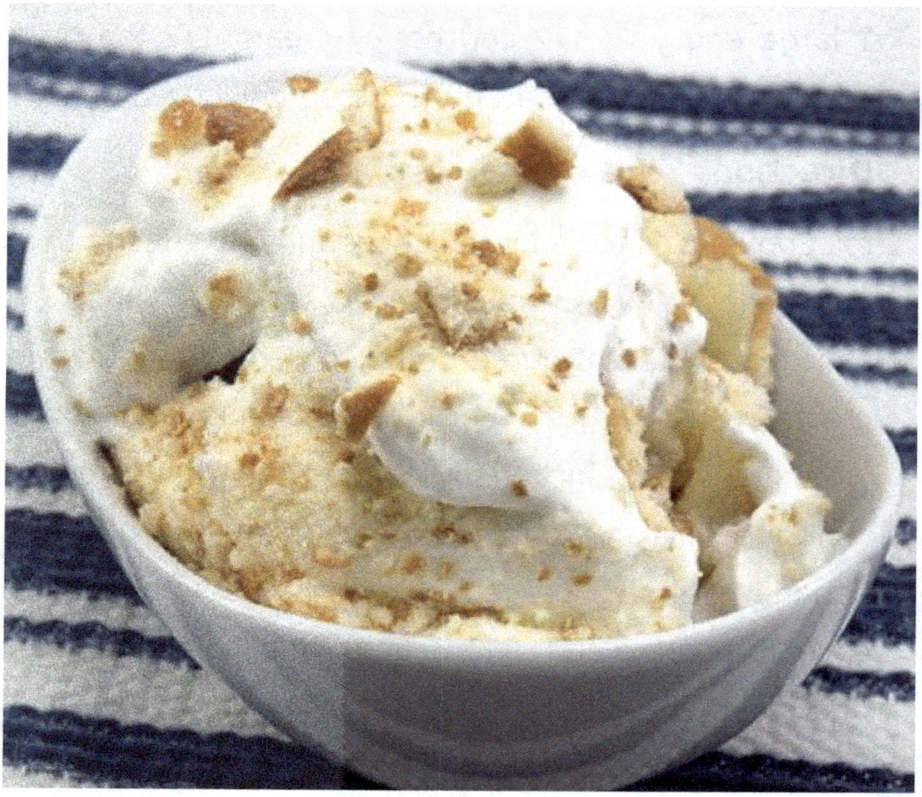

Green Tea Mug Cake

Servings:1 Preparation Time: 12 Minutes

Ingredients:

1 large egg 1 tbsp coconut oil 1 tsp baking powder 1 pinch sea salt 2 tbsp frozen sugar-free white chocolate chips, frozen ½ tsp vanilla extract ½ tspmatcha powder ¼ cup almond flour 1/8 tsp xanthan gum 5-10 drops liquid stevia 1 ½ tbsp powdered erythritol

Directions

for Cooking: Lightly grease the inside of a mug with cooking spray and preheat oven to 350oF. In a small bowl, whisk well egg, coconut oil, baking powder, salt, vanilla, and liquid stevia. Stir in matcha powder, almond flour, xanthan gum, and erythritol. Mix well. Fold in frozen white choco chips. Transfer to prepared mug. Pop in the oven and bake for 12 minutes. Let cool a bit and enjoy.

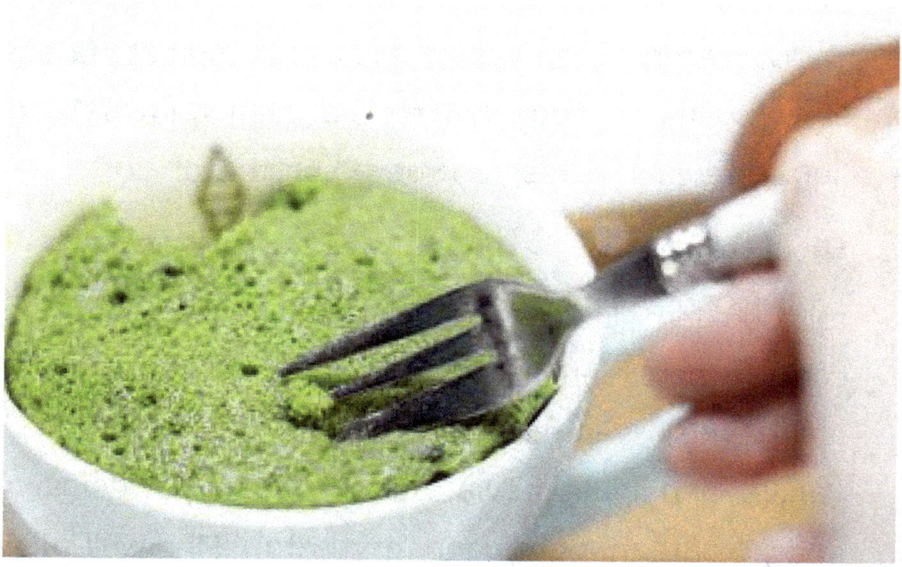

Brownie Muffin Approved

Servings:6 Preparation Time: 30 Minutes

Ingredients:

¼ cup cocoa powder ¼ cup slivered almonds ¼ cup sugar-free caramel syrup ½ cup pumpkin puree ½ tablespoon baking powder ½ teaspoon salt 1 cup golden flaxseed meal 1 large egg 1 tablespoon cinnamon 1 teaspoon apple cider vinegar 1 teaspoon vanilla extract 2 tablespoons coconut oil

Directions

for Cooking: Line six muffin tins with muffin liners and preheat oven to 350oF. In a large mixing bowl, whisk well egg and salt. Whisk in caramel syrup, baking powder, pumpkin puree, cinnamon, apple cider, vanilla extract, and coconut oil. Mix thoroughly. Add cocoa powder and flaxseed meal. Mix well. Evenly divide batter into prepared muffin tins and sprinkle almonds on top. Pop in the oven and bake for 15 minutes. Cool and enjoy.

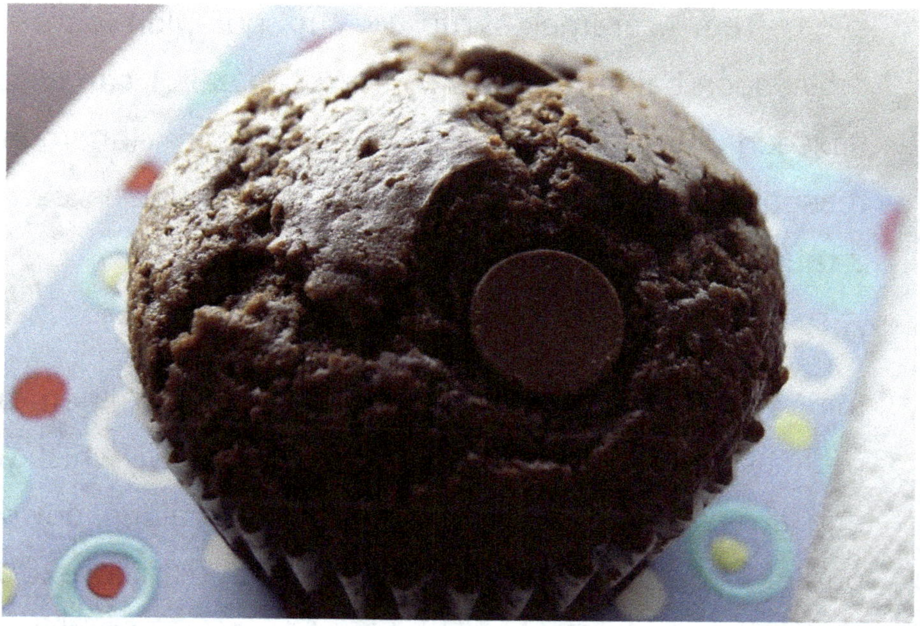

Fruity Smoothie

Preparation Time: 10 minutes Cooking Time: 0 minute

Servings: 1

Ingredients:

¾ cup plain yogurt ½ cup pineapple juice 1 cup pineapple chunks 1 cup raspberries, sliced 1 cup blueberries, sliced

Direction:

Process the ingredients in a blender. Chill before serving.

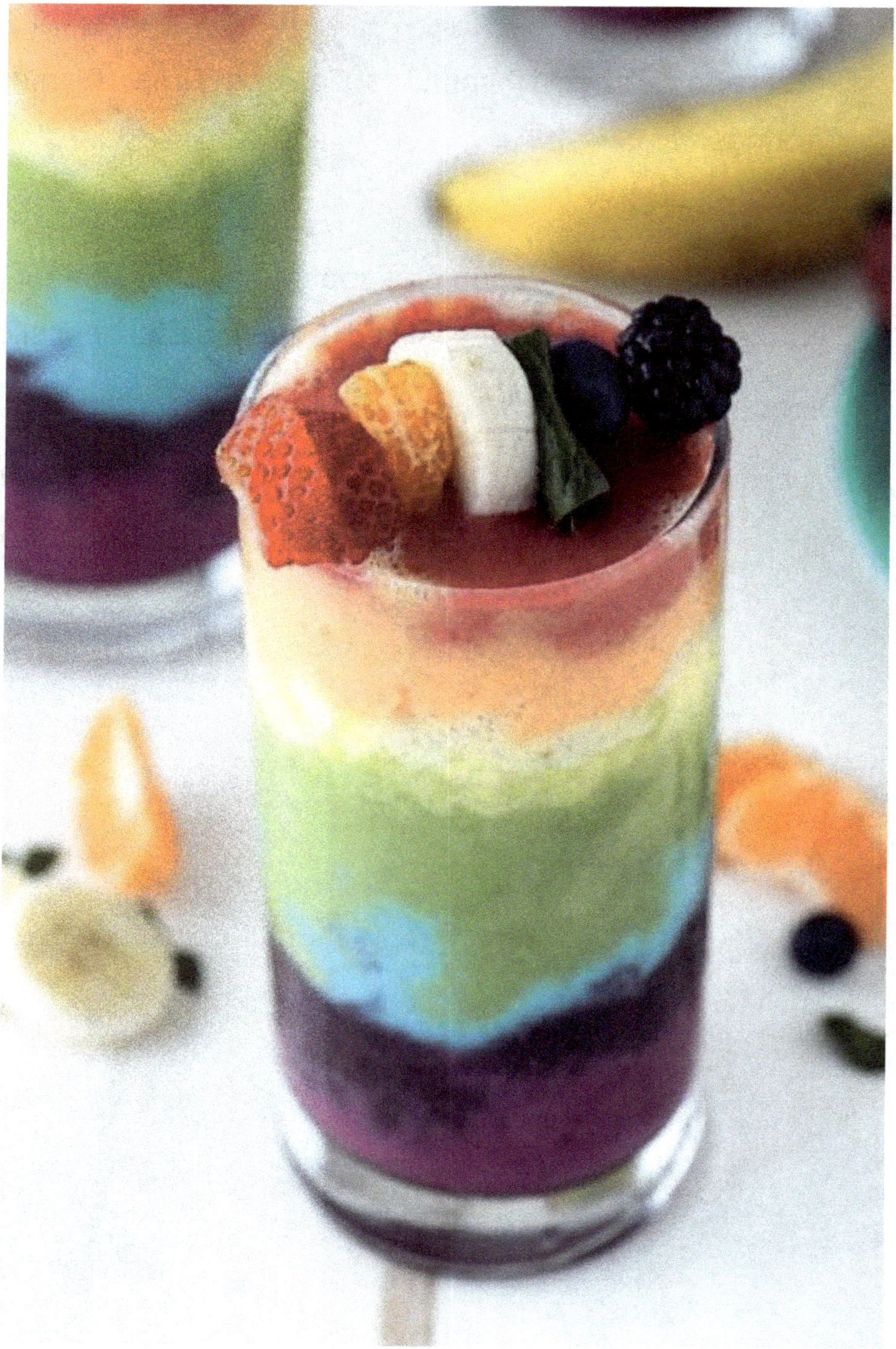

Lemon Drink

Servings: 12 Preparation time: 2 hours and 10 minutes

Ingredients:

1 cinnamon stick, about 3 inches long 1/2 teaspoon of whole cloves 2 cups of coconut sugar 4 fluid of ounce pineapple juice 1/2 cup and 2 tablespoons of lemon juice 12 fluid ounce of orange juice 2 1/2 quarts of water

Directions:

Pour water into a 6-quarts slow cooker and stir the sugar and lemon juice properly. Wrap the cinnamon, the whole cloves in cheesecloth and tie its corners with string. Immerse this cheesecloth bag in the liquid present in the slow cooker and cover it with the lid. Then plug in the slow cooker and let it cook on high heat setting for 2 hours or until it is heated thoroughly. When done, discard the cheesecloth bag and serve the drink hot or cold.

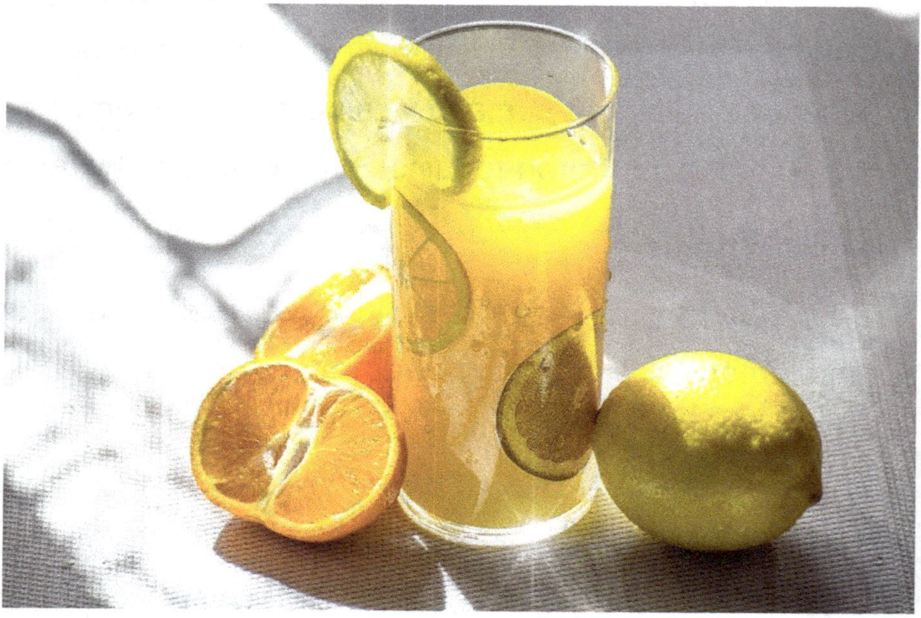

Nice Spiced Cherry Cider

Servings: 16 Preparation time: 4 hours and 5 minutes

Ingredients:

2 cinnamon sticks, each about 3 inches long 6-ounce of cherry gelatin 4 quarts of apple cider

Directions:

Using a 6-quarts slow cooker, pour the apple cider and add the cinnamon stick. Stir, then cover the slow cooker with its lid. Plug in the cooker and let it cook for 3 hours at the high heat setting or until it is heated thoroughly. Then add and stir the gelatin properly, then continue cooking for another hour. When done, remove the cinnamon sticks and serve the drink hot or cold.

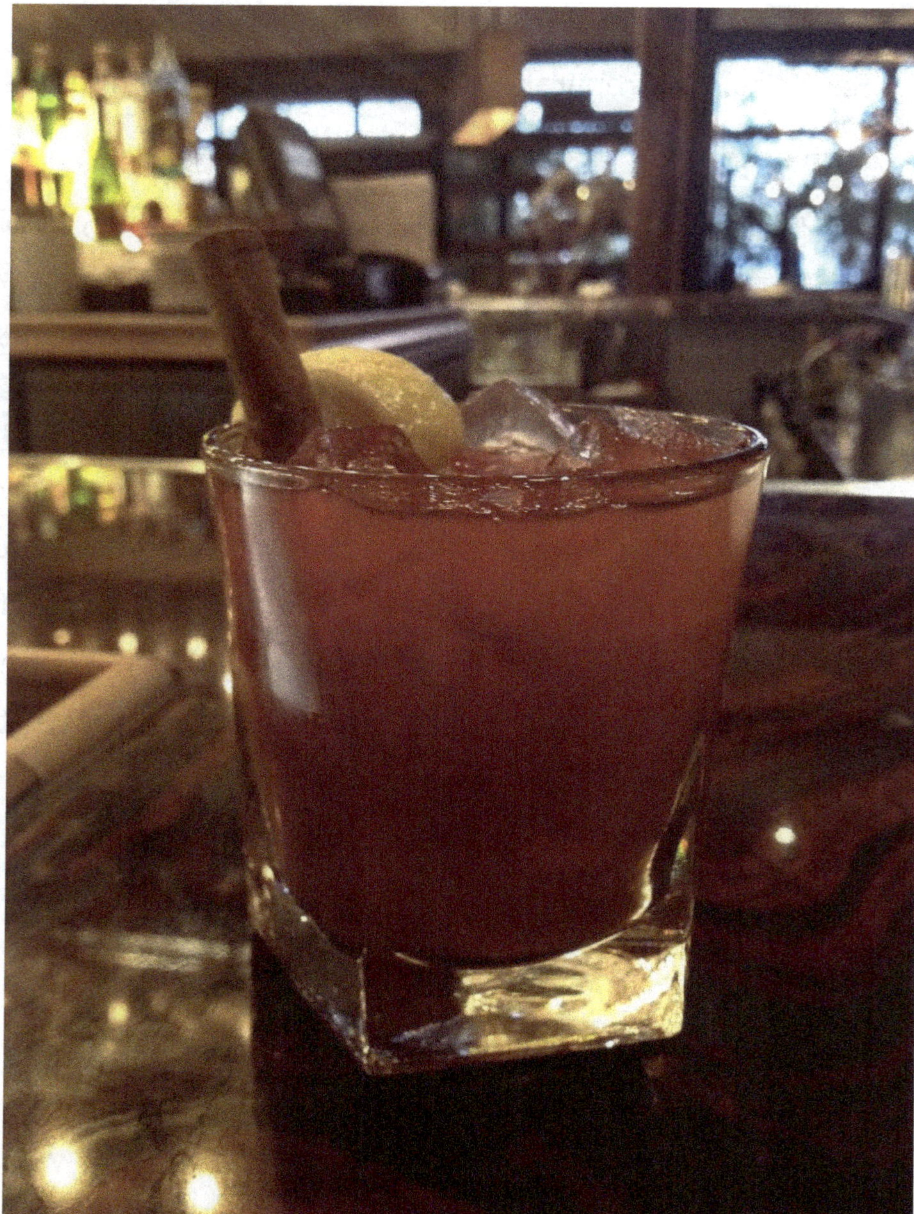

Tangy Spiced Cranberry Drink

Servings: 14 Preparation time: 2 hours and 10 minutes

Ingredients:

1 1/2 cups of coconut sugar 12 whole cloves 2 fluid ounce of lemon juice 6 fluid ounce of orange juice 32 fluid ounce of cranberry juice 8 cups of hot water 1/2 cup of Red Hot candies

Directions:

Pour the water into a 6-quarts slow cooker along with the cranberry juice, orange juice, and the lemon juice. Stir the sugar properly. Wrap the whole cloves in a cheese cloth, tie its corners with strings, and immerse it in the liquid present inside the slow cooker. Add the red-hot candies to the slow cooker and cover it with the lid. Then plug in the slow cooker and let it cook on the low heat setting for 3 hours or until it is heated thoroughly. When done, discard the cheesecloth bag and serve.

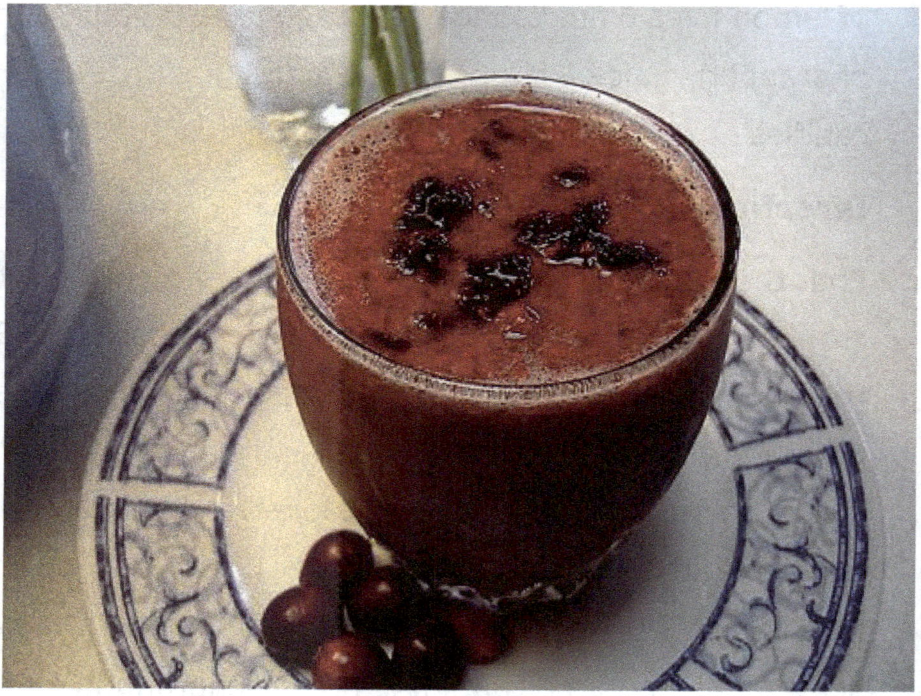

Coffee Mousse

Preparation time: 5 minutesCooking time: 40 minutes

Servings: 2

Ingredients:

2 packages (2 Tbs.) unflavored gelatin 1½ cups confectioners' sugar 2 egg whites 2 cups heavy cream 1 cup milk 6 Tbs. triple-strength espresso ¼ tsp. cinnamon ½ cup cold water 1 oz. shaved bittersweet chocolate

Directions:

Combine the sugar and the milk in a medium-sized saucepan and heat it over a medium flame, stirring constantly, until all the sugar is dissolved. Stir in the espresso and the cinnamon. Dissolve the gelatin in the cold water and then stir it into the milk. Heat the mixture until the gelatin is completely dissolved, then remove it from the heat and allow it to cool, stirring occasionally. Beat the egg whites until they hold stiff peaks, and in a separate bowl whip the cream until stiff. As soon as the cooled gelatin mixture begins to thicken, stir in the whipped cream and fold in the beaten egg whites. Pile the mousse into 6 or 8 individual dessert dishes, decorate it with the shaved chocolate, and chill it for about 2 hours before serving.

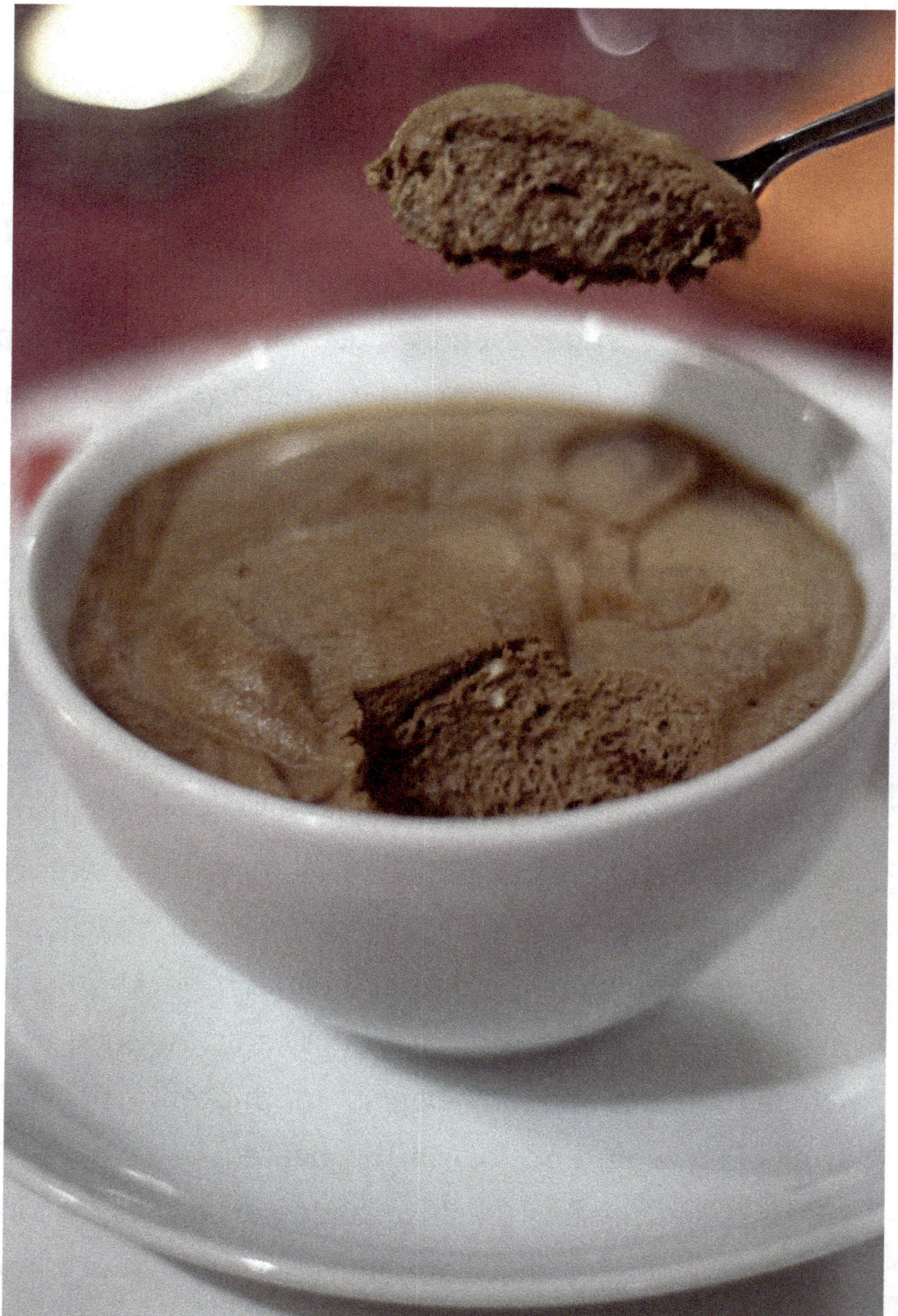

Yellow Squash Puffs

Preparation time: 5 minutesCooking time: 30 minutes Servings: 2

Ingredients:

1 medium onion, grated 1 tsp baking powder 1/3 cup all-purpose flour 1 cup yellow squash, cooked and mashed ½ tsp salt 1/3 cup cornmeal 1 egg, beaten

Directions:

Mix the egg and cooked squash. Toss to combine. Combine the baking salt, cornmeal, flour and salt in a large bowl. Add the squash mixture. Stir to combine. Add the onions. Drop a tablespoon full of the mixture into the hot oil. Cook until it is golden brown. Turn it occasionally to ensure that it is cooked on all sides. Place on paper towels to drain excess oil.

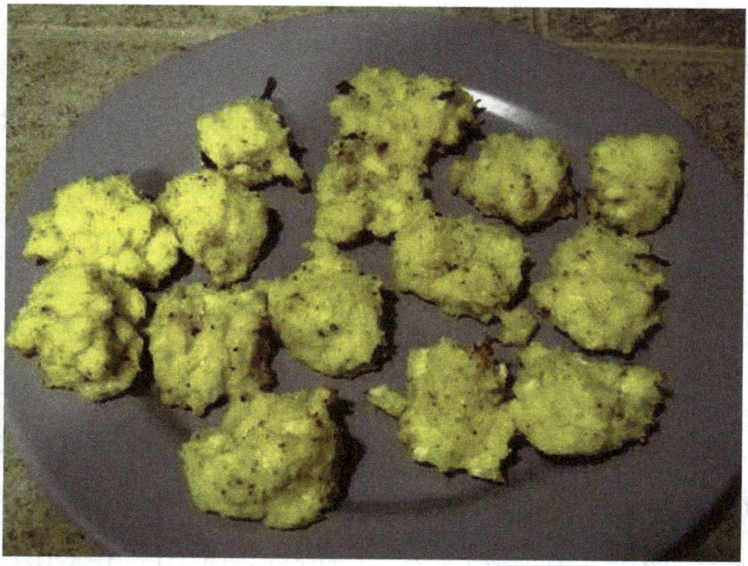

Vibrant Lemon Millet Cookies

Preparation time: 15 minutes Cooking time: 65 minutes

20 cookies.

Ingredients:

1/3 cup olive oil 5 tbsp. vegan yogurt zest from 3 lemons juice from 1 lemon 1 cup flour ½ cup brown sugar ½ cup oats ½ cup millet flakes ½ cup unsweetened coconut flakes

Directions:

Begin by preheating the oven to 400 degrees Fahrenheit. Next, mix together the dry and wet ingredients separately, and then bring the two mixtures together. Next, roll the cookies into twenty balls and place them on a baking sheet. Bake the cookies for fifteen minutes, and enjoy.

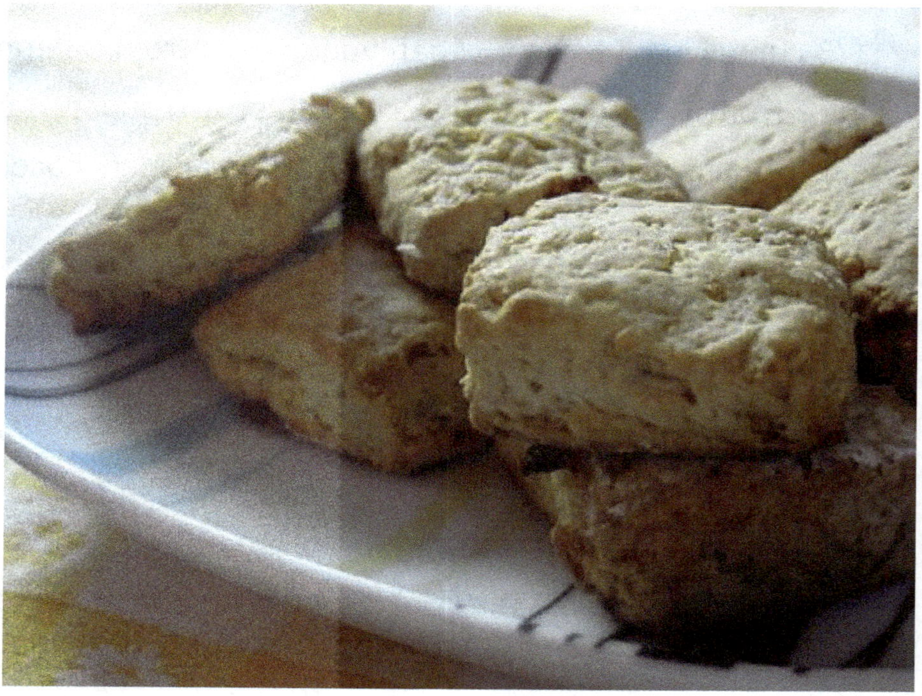

Vegan Pumpkin and Chocolate Pie

Preparation time: 15 minutes Cooking time: 45 minutes 12 slices.

Ingredients:

1 cup canned pumpkin ½ cup coconut oil 1 cup cane sugar 1 cup all-purpose flour 1 tbsp. cornstarch 1 ½ tsp. vanilla 1 tsp. salt ½ cup cocoa powder 1 tsp. baking soda Pumpkin Layer Ingredients: 1 cup canned pumpkin 1 tsp. vanilla 2 tbsp. arrowroot 4 tbsp. almond milk 1/3 cup cane sugar 2 tsp. cinnamon ½ tsp. ginger ½ tsp. nutmeg

Directions: Begin by preheating your oven to 350 degrees Fahrenheit. Next, mix together the canned pumpkin puree, the coconut oil, the cane sugar, the flour, the cornstarch, the vanilla, the salt, the cocoa powder, and the baking soda. Spread this mixture to the bottom of the pie plate. Next, mix together the ingredients from the pumpkin pie layer. Add this mixture overtop the first layer. Bake the vegan pie in the preheated oven for forty minutes. Allow the pie to cool and chill in the fridge prior to serving. Enjoy!

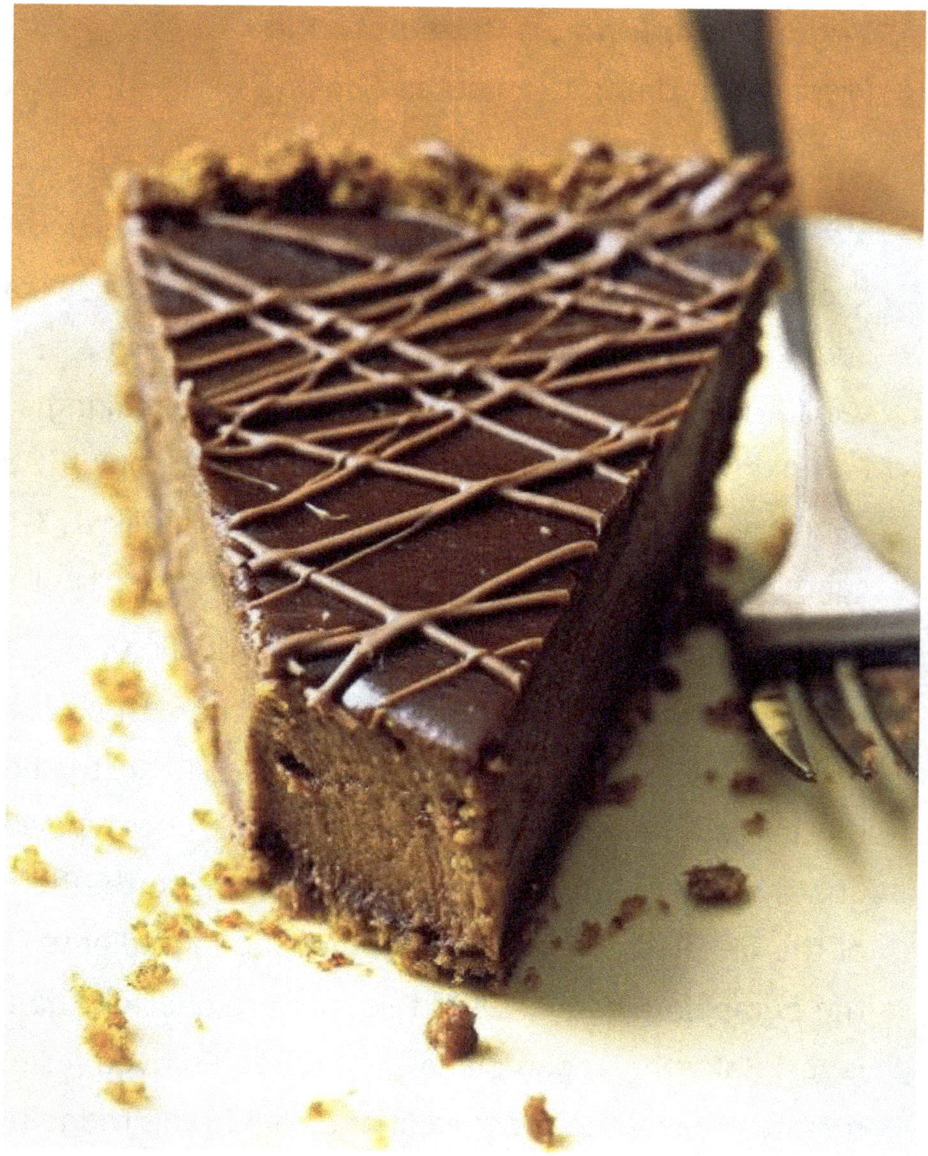

Very Blueberry Morning Coffee Cake

Preparation time: 15 minutes Cooking time: 25 minutes 9 Servings.

Ingredients:

1 ¼ cup whole-wheat flour 1 tsp. baking powder ¼ tsp. baking soda ¾ cup sugar ¼ cup applesauce ½ cup soymilk 3 tbsp. vegan butter 1 tsp. vanilla 1 tbsp. apple cider vinegar ½ tsp. almond extract 1 cup frozen blueberries 2 tbsp. brown sugar ½ tsp. cinnamon

Directions: Begin by preheating your oven to 350 degrees Fahrenheit. Next, mix together the brown sugar and the cinnamon. Melt the vegan butter in a microwave during this time, as well. Mix together the dry ingredients in a large mixing bowl. Next, add the melted butter, the almond milk, the vinegar, the extracts, and the applesauce. Stir well, and allow the dry ingredients to become moistened. Add the blueberries last. Pour the ingredients into a cake pan, and spread the brown sugar and cinnamon overtop the cake. Bake the cake for thirty minutes, and allow it to cool. Enjoy.

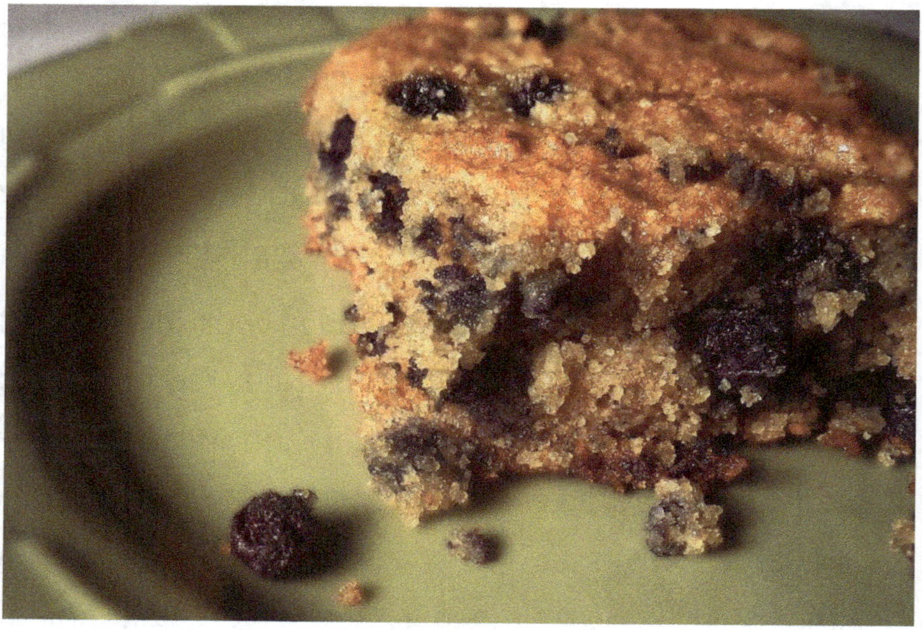

Vegan-Inspired Coconut Cake

Preparation time: 15 minutes Cooking time: 25 minutes 8 slices.

Ingredients:

2 cups shredded coconut 3 cups almond milk 2 tsp. apple cider vinegar 3 tsp. flax meal 1 cup toasted coconut flour 2 cups all-purpose flour 1 tsp. baking soda 4 tsp. baking powder 1 cup coconut sugar 2 tsp. vanilla ½ cup coconut oil 1 tsp. salt

Directions:

Begin by preheating your oven to 375 degrees Fahrenheit. Next, mix together the almond milk, the flax meal, and the apple cider vinegar. Push this to the side. In a different bowl, stir together the coconut flour, the bread flour, the baking powder, and the baking soda. Next, mix together the coconut oil, the coconut sugar, the vanilla, and the salt. Add all the ingredients together in a large bowl, and stir well. Pour the created batter in two cake pans and bake the cakes for thirty minutes. Allow the cakes to cool prior to frosting them with your favorite vegan frosting. Enjoy.

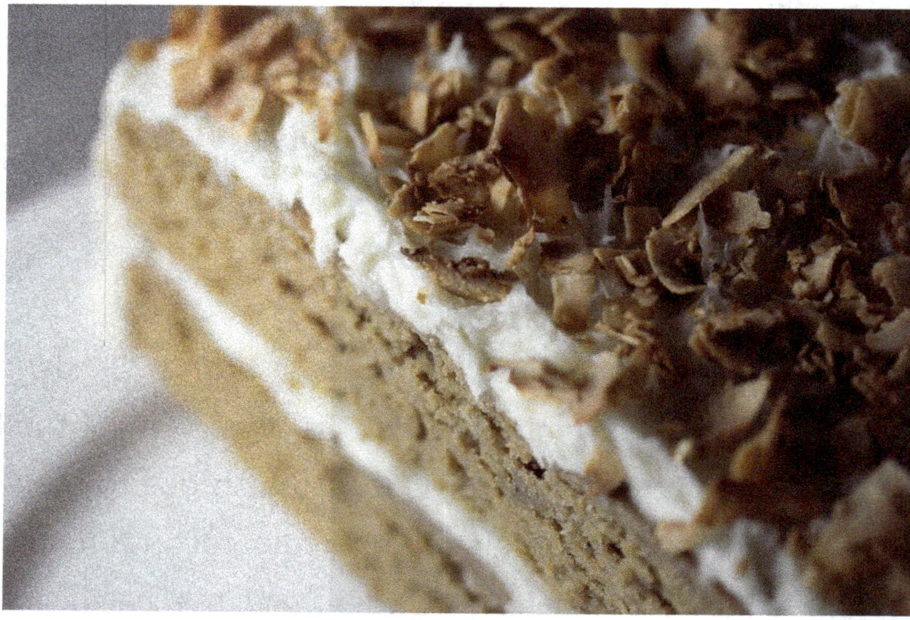

Apricot and Chocolate Scones

Preparation time: 5 minutesCooking time: 50 minutes Servings: 2

Ingredients:

1/3 cup white vanilla baking chips 1/4 teaspoon salt 1/3 cup butter 2 teaspoons baking powder 1 and 3/4 cups all-purpose flour 1/4 cup sugar 1 egg 1/3 cup dried apricots Shortening (for greasing cookie sheet) Half and half

Directions

For the Dough Preheat your oven to 400 degrees F. In a medium-sized bowl, mix 2 teaspoons baking powder, 1 and 3/4 cups all-purpose flour, 1/4 cup sugar and 1/4 teaspoon salt. Use a pastry blend to cut the firm butter until it turns into crumbs. In a small bowl, pour 1/3 cup white vanilla baking chips and set it aside to melt in normal room temperature. Lightly dust a baking sheet with flour and knead the dough mixture. Slice the dough into eight wedges and bake in the oven for 16 minutes. For the Scones Dough Grease your cookie sheet lightly with shortening and set aside. In the same bowl, add apricots, half and half, baking chips and 1 egg. If you do not have access to ready-made half and half, you can mix 4 parts of whole milk with 1 part of heavy cream. Once the dough is done, remove the cookie sheet and slice the scones. Place the melted white vanilla baking chips in a plastic bag and turn it into a makeshift icing pipe bag. Arrange the scones and pipe over the vanilla chips as frosting. Garnish the scones with apricots and serve warm on a plate.

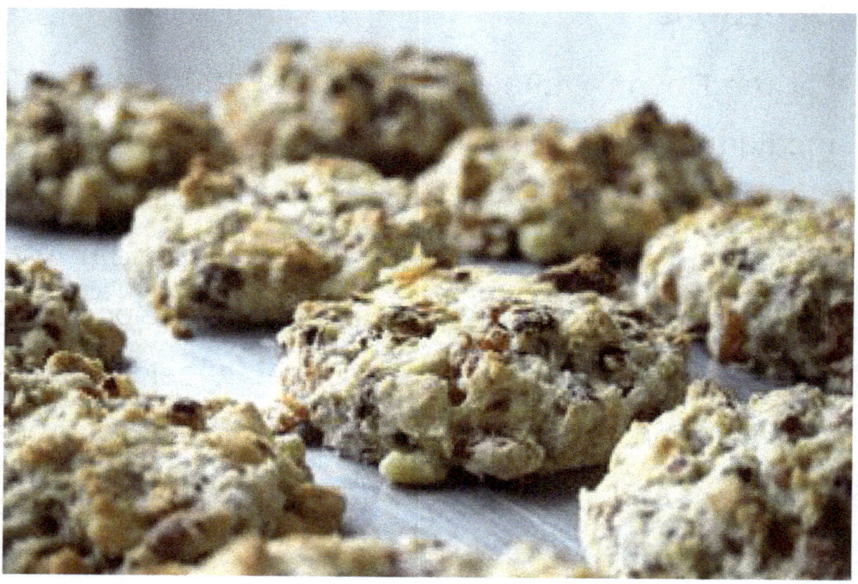

Lemon-Cream Cheese Scones

Preparation time: 5 minutesCooking time: 45 minutes

Servings: 2

Ingredients:

2 teaspoons baking powder 1/4 cup sugar 1/3 cup firm butter 2 and 1/4 cups all-purpose flour 1 tablespoon lemon peels or dehydrated lemon zest 1/3 cup milk Lemon juice 1/4 teaspoon salt Sugar 1 package cream cheese 1 egg

Directions:

Preheat the oven to 400 degrees F. In a large bowl, mix salt, baking powder, sugar and dehydrated lemon zest. Use a pastry blender to slice the firm butter into crumbs. In a small bowl, mix the eggs, milk and cream cheese with the flour mixture. In an ungreased cookie sheet, place 8 dough balls brushed with sugar and lemon juice. Bake the dough in the oven for 18 minutes and peel them off the cookie sheet once done. Serve the Light and Flaky Lemon-Cream Cheese Scones on a plate and enjoy the sinful treat!

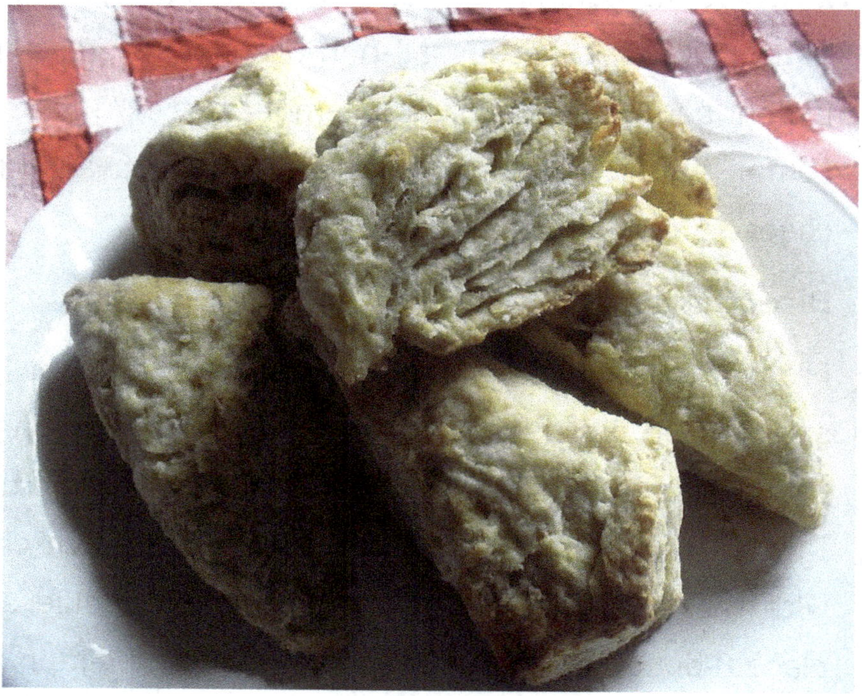

Raspberry Chia Smoothie

Preparation time: 30 minutes Cooking time: 0 minutes Servings: 01

Ingredients:

¾ cup of almond milk 1 cup raspberries ½ of a banana 1 tablespoon chia seeds ½ of an avocado 2 handful of spinach Ice for thickness

Directions:

Add all the ingredients to a blender. Hit the pulse button and blend till it is smooth. Chill well and garnish as desired. Serve.

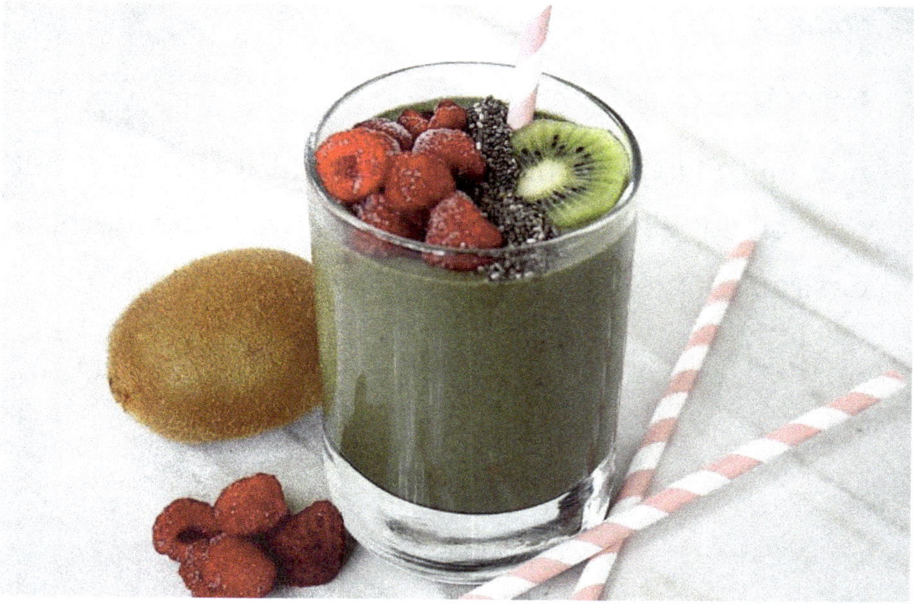

Mango Carrot Smoothie

Preparation time: 30 minutes Cooking time: 0 minutes Servings: 01

Ingredients:

1 cup carrots, chopped 1 cup frozen mango 1 cup frozen pineapple 1 cup frozen strawberries ¼ cup soy yogurt ½ cup soy milk 1 tablespoon chia seeds

Directions:

Add all the ingredients to a blender. Hit the pulse button and blend till it is smooth. Chill well to serve.

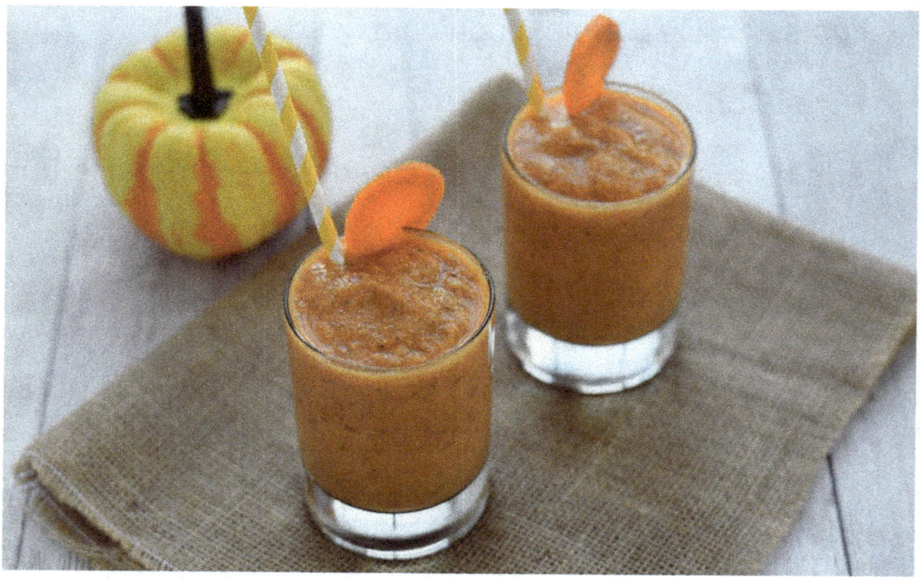

Blueberry Peach Tea Smoothie

Preparation time: 30 minutes Cooking time: 0 minutes Servings: 01

Ingredients:

1 cup black tea, brewed and cooled 5.3 ounces soy yogurt 1 cup blueberries ½ cup peaches Ice

Directions:

Add all ingredients to a blender. Hit the pulse button and blend till it is smooth. Chill well to serve.

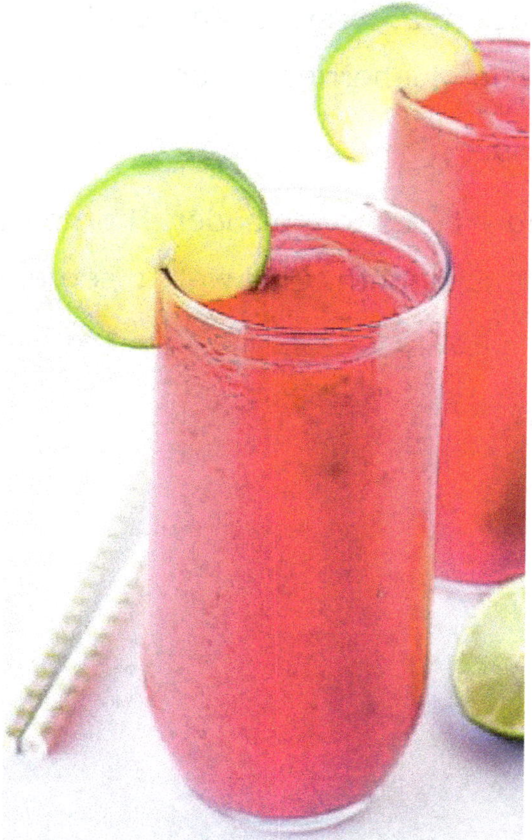

MCT Green Smoothie

Preparation time: 30 minutes Cooking time: 0 minutes

Servings: 01

Ingredients:

1 ½ cups ice 1 banana 2 handfuls of spinach ½ avocado

2 cups almond milk 2 scoops plant-based protein powder

1 tablespoon MCT oil

Directions: Add all ingredients to a blender. Hit the pulse button and blend till it is smooth. Chill well to serve.

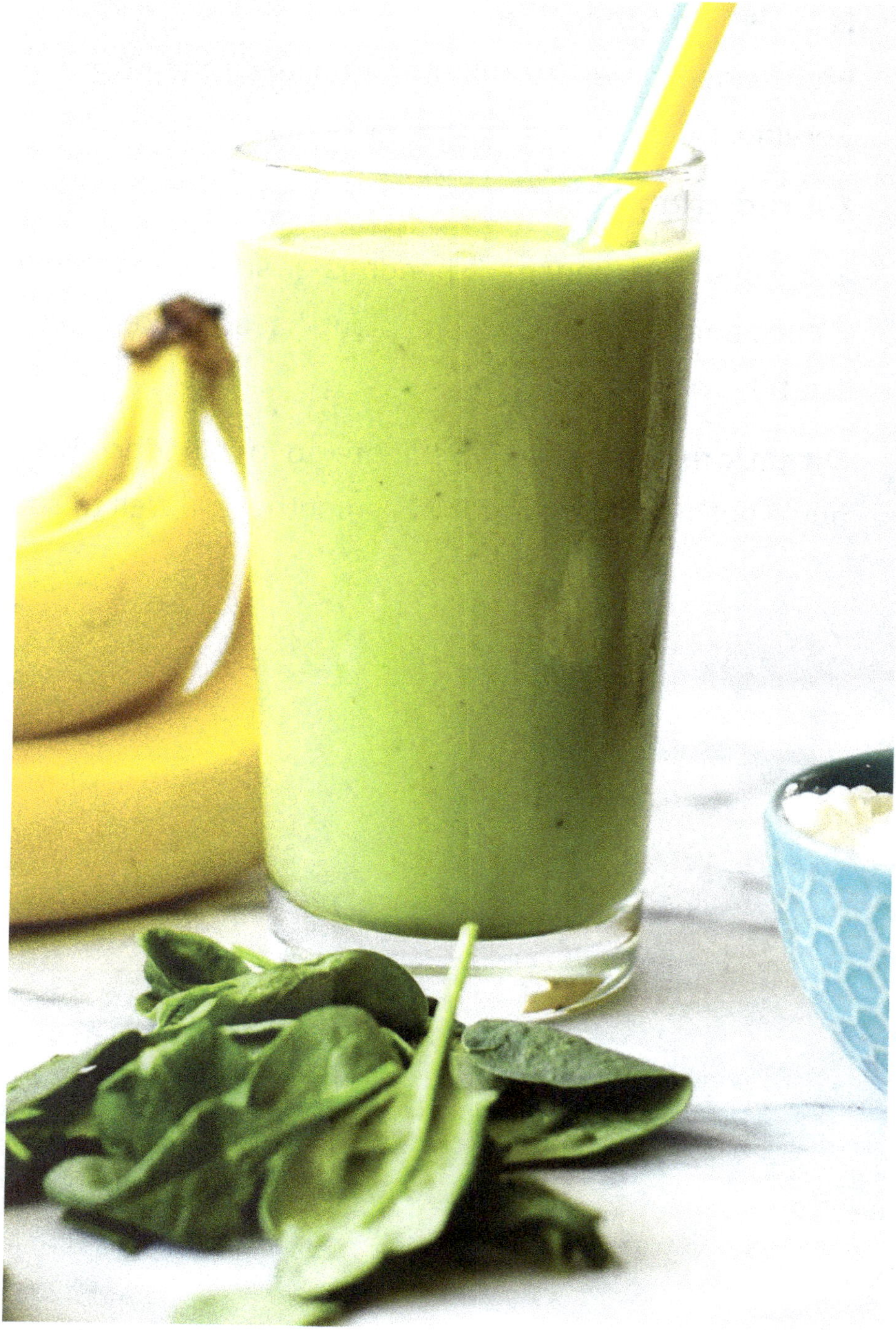

CPSIA information can be obtained
at www.ICGtesting.com
Printed in the USA
LVHW081656250521
688475LV00008B/572

9 781802 696806